An International Collection of Unique Aerosol Cans

国际特色
气雾罐荟萃

主编◎游一中　周润峰

摄影◎王星际　张伟新

U0397382

东南大学出版社
SOUTHEAST UNIVERSITY PRESS
·南京·

内容简介

本书以近50年来收集到的国际特色铝和马口铁气雾罐为主体,计有205只铝气雾罐和59只马口铁气雾罐,采用中英文介绍、图片和360度旋转视频等方式展示各罐的特点。其中,大部分是2008—2024年参加欧洲国际铝气雾罐竞赛的参赛样品,马口铁气雾罐是历次国际气雾剂展览会收集到的样品。

本书的收集数量和类型,为国内外首次,以文字、图片和360度旋转视频介绍这么多气雾罐在国内外也尚属首次。

要想了解本书收集的所有气雾罐的全貌,可通过手机扫二维码观看360度旋转视频。

图书在版编目(CIP)数据

国际特色气雾罐荟萃 / 游一中,周润峰主编.
南京 : 东南大学出版社,2024. 12. -- ISBN 978-7
-5766-1675-0

Ⅰ. R944.7-49

中国国家版本馆 CIP 数据核字第 202467GC37 号

策划编辑:张丽萍 责任编辑:陈 佳 责任校对:周 菊 封面设计:毕 真 责任印制:周荣虎

国际特色气雾罐荟萃
GUOJI TESE QIWUGUAN HUICUI

主　　编:游一中　周润峰
出版发行:东南大学出版社
社　　址:南京市四牌楼 2 号　　邮编:210096　　电话:025-83793330
出 版 人:白云飞
网　　址:http://www.seupress.com
电子邮箱:press@seupress.com
经　　销:全国各地新华书店
印　　刷:江阴金马印刷有限公司
开　　本:787 mm×1 092 mm　1/16
印　　张:13
字　　数:411 千
版　　次:2024 年 12 月第 1 版
印　　次:2024 年 12 月第 1 次印刷
书　　号:ISBN 978-7-5766-1675-0
定　　价:128.00 元

前　言

　　气雾罐是储存气雾剂的容器。它耐压密闭，与内容物接触及在环境中均耐腐蚀。其使用操作方便，外形美观。无论是材质选取、制罐过程，还是回收环节均符合环保要求。

　　本书收集了2008—2024年间参加国际铝气雾罐竞赛的205只样品罐，涵盖每只气雾罐的参赛资料、图片及360度旋转视频，旨在让读者全方位了解每只气雾罐的特色。书中还罗列了作者历经数十载在世界各国精心搜集到的特色马口铁气雾罐59只，并配有图片和360度旋转视频。

　　这些颇具特色的气雾罐，既反映了人们应用思路的变迁，又体现了罐体设计、制罐技术有了新的改进，还折射出人们非凡的审美价值。倘若您能发现每只罐的特色并找出它具有特色的原因，那么祝贺您，这意味着您对气雾罐的了解已然更进一层。

　　期望本书能为您在生产和应用更优的气雾罐时拓宽眼界，打开思路，此乃我们共同的愿望！

目 录

1

第一篇
国际特色铝气雾罐

一、2024 年国际铝气雾罐竞赛参赛罐

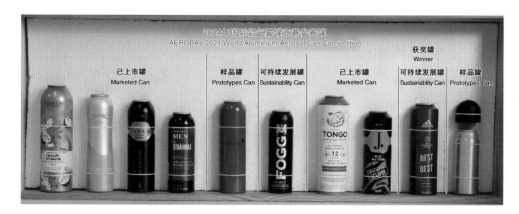

产品编号从左至右分别是:7,2,3A,1,4,6,9,3B,8,5

编号:2024-1

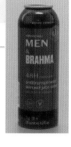

英文介绍

Can No. 1: O Boticário Men Antiperspirant Deodorant

Marketed Can

Description: This aerosol uses a 45 mm×130 mm can with a round shoulder. It contains the manufacturer's proprietary alloy blend, which uses up to 25% recycled content. The can is designed for the celebration of Father's Day.

中文介绍

1 号罐:

已上市罐

产品说明:

这款气雾剂使用 45 mm×130 mm 的圆肩罐。它含有制造商专有的合金混合物,其中含有高达 25% 的再生材料。该气雾罐是为了庆祝父亲节而设计的。

2024-1 号罐 360 度旋转视频二维码

编号：2024-2

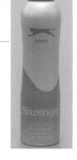

英文介绍

Can No. 2: Slazenger Women's Deodorant

Marketed Can

Description: This new aerosol can, crafted in dimensions of 45 mm×158 mm, boasts a distinctive pearlescent enamel base and a semi-matte finish. It stands out with its shape, size, and ergonomic design. With attractive fragrances and color options, the products have already found their place on the shelves and have gained popularity among the intended target consumers.

中文介绍

2 号罐：

已上市罐

产品说明：

这款新的气雾剂罐尺寸为 45 mm×158 mm，采用珠光底涂层和半哑光油，以其形状、尺寸和符合人体工程学的设计脱颖而出。该产品凭借诱人的香味和多种色彩选择已经成功上架，并受到了目标消费者的欢迎。

2024-2 号罐 360 度旋转视频二维码

编号：2024-3A

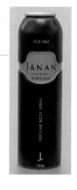

英文介绍

Can No. 3A: J. "JANAN" Body Spray

Marketed Can

Description: This can (50 mm×150 mm, with a half-moon embossing) is created for the new perfume body spray collection of J. Junaid Jamshed Privated Limited Company, which is the biggest perfume producer in Pakistan. For their premium body spray project, the company is seeking an innovative solution.

After a long study on the aluminium can type, the customer opts for the manufacturer's innovative technology called "360° Embossed Shaping with Oriented Printing". The type of the embossed shape is half moon and the brand JANAN has been highlighted on it. Thanks to this technology, the brand stands out against other brands on the market.

中 文 介 绍

3A 号罐：

已上市罐

产品说明：

这种铝罐（50 mm×150 mm，半月浮雕）是为巴基斯坦最大的香水生产商 J. Junaid Jamshed 私人有限公司的新香水身体喷雾系列而设计的。对于他们的高端身体喷雾项目，该公司想要一个创新的解决方案。

在对铝罐类型进行了长时间的研究后，客户决定采用制造商的创新技术"360°浮雕成型与定向印刷"。浮雕形状为半月形，上面突显了 JANAN 品牌。得益于这项技术，该品牌能够在市场上脱颖而出。

2024-3A 号罐 360 度旋转视频二维码

编号：2024-3B

英 文 介 绍

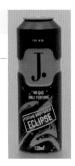

Can No. 3B: J. "No Gas, Only Perfume" Body Spray

Marketed Can

Description: This can (45 mm×135 mm, with a square embossing) is created for J. Junaid Jamshed Privated Limited Company. For their premium men's no-gas perfume in aluminium can, J. company requires an innovative aluminium can solution to their new no-gas perfume projects.

The customer chooses the manufacturer's innovative technology called "360° Embossed Shaping with Oriented Printing" for this can. The type of the embossed shape is square and the brand "J." has been highlighted on the square embossed shape.

As the artworks of the men's no-gas perfume range have been designed with attractive colors and designs for the different models (ENIGMA, VELOCITY, ECLIPSE, EXODUS), the can has been successful in capturing the consumers' attention.

中 文 介 绍

3B 号罐：

已上市罐

产品说明：

这款铝罐（45 mm×135 mm，方形浮雕）是为 J. Junaid Jamshed 私人有限公司设计的。对于其高端男士无气体香水，该公司需要一个创新的铝罐解决方案。

客户选择了制造商称为"360°浮雕成型与定向印刷"的创新技术。浮雕形状为方形,方形浮雕上突出了"J"品牌。

由于男士无气体香水系列铝罐采用了具有吸引力的颜色,并且针对不同款型(ENIGMA, VELOCITY, ECLIPSE, EXODUS)分别进行设计,已经成功吸引了消费者的注意。

2024-3B 号罐 360 度旋转视频二维码

编号:2024-4

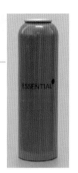

英文介绍

Can No. 4: ESSENTIAL—Special Effect Overcoat

Prototypes Can

Description: Normally, the over varnish is clear to protect the decoration of the can. However, this can has been decorated with a newly developed over varnish that gives a unique finish. It is a decorative element and enhances the minimalist design by incorporating gold pigments into the over varnish. By adding just 1%-2% of effect pigments to the formula of the varnish, a stunning effect can be achieved, making the can stand out at the point of sale against the other "normal" cans, showcasing a full body decoration with a reasonable cost.

This development is easily adaptable to industrial production and does not limit necking options. It has no adverse effects on the curing, washing or any other processes during manufacturing.

中文介绍

4 号罐:

样品罐

产品说明:

通常情况下,铝罐的光油是透明的,以保护罐子的表面印刷效果。然而,这款罐体采用了一种新研发的光油,具有独特的饰面效果。它是一种装饰元素,通过在光油中加入金色颜料,增强了极简主义设计的效果。只在光油中加入 1%~2% 的特效颜料,就能达到令人惊艳的效果,使该罐体在销售点与其他"常规"罐子一同展出时能脱颖而出,而且成本合理。

这种技术很容易适应工业化生产,而且不存在肩型选择限制。在生产过程中,它对固化、洗涤或其他工艺都没有不利影响。

2024-4 号罐 360 度旋转视频二维码

编号:2024-5

英 文 介 绍

Can No. 5: Next Gen Can

Prototypes Can

Description: This can has an innovative segment thread and a matching screw cap. This ground-breaking solution sets new standards in terms of safety, user-friendliness, and sustainability. With the standardized 1-inch opening, the can is perfectly compatible with established accessories such as spray nozzles and valves. The clever segment thread facilitates the simple and secure attachment of the screw cap, which prevents unintentional spread of the contents—neither during transportation nor in daily use. Even if hit by a strong force during transport, the resistant screw cap reliably protects the contents and at the same time prevents the spray nozzle from being unintentionally triggered. The seal also protects against moisture and dust, ideal for special applications.

Thanks to the special segment thread, it can be used effortlessly with dispensers and special adapters. Flexible and versatile, they adapt to individual requirements in the cosmetics, pharmaceutical, personal care, household, and industrial sectors.

中 文 介 绍

5 号罐:

样品罐

产品说明:

该罐具有创新的分段螺纹和与之匹配的螺旋盖。这一突破性的解决方案在安全性、用户友好性和可持续性方面树立了新的标准。标准化的 1 英寸口径,可以完美地与既定的配件如喷嘴和阀门兼容。巧妙的分段螺纹使得螺旋盖的连接简单安全,无论是在运输过程中还是在日常使用中,都可以防止内容物的意外泄露。即使在运输过程中受到强力撞击,耐用的螺旋盖也能可靠地保护内容物,同时防止喷嘴被意外触发。密封件也防潮防尘,非常适合特殊应用。

由于特殊的分段螺纹设计,它很容易与分配器和特殊适配器一起使用。设计的灵活性和多功能,使得它们适用于化妆品、制药、个人护理、家庭和工业部门的个性化需求。

2024-5 号罐 360 度旋转视频二维码

编号：2024-6

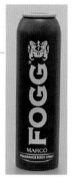

英文介绍

Can No. 6: Fogg Deodorant

Sustainability Can

Description: A collaboration with VINI International makes Fogg deodorant stand out due to its innovative use of a special metered pump valve system. Unlike traditional pressurized cans, which rely on propellant gases to disperse the deodorant, Fogg's cans dispense the product in a controlled manner. This method not only eliminates the need for propellant gases but also ensures precise application, minimizing waste, with each spray delivering the exact amount needed, avoiding the common issue of over-spraying and ensuring that the deodorant is used efficiently. The elimination of propellant gases reduces greenhouse gas emissions and also simplifies the manufacturing process, as there is no need to pressurize the containers. This streamlining of production not only lowers energy consumption but also results in cost savings, making the product economically viable without compromising on environmental responsibility.

A key sustainability element is the use of aluminium cans. The recyclability of aluminium ensures that the packaging can be reused indefinitely, aligning perfectly with the company's sustainability goals.

中文介绍

6 号罐：

可持续发展罐

产品说明：

与 VINI 国际合作,使得 Fogg 香体剂因创新使用一种特殊计量泵阀系统而脱颖而出。与依靠推进剂气体分散香体剂的传统加压罐不同,Fogg 的罐以可控的方式进行给料。这种方法不仅消除了对推进剂气体的需求,而且确保了精确的应用,最大限度地减少了浪费,每次喷雾都能提供所需的精确量,避免了过度喷洒的常见问题,并确保了香体剂的有效使用。因为不需要对容器加压,推进剂气体的取消减少了温室气体的排放,也简化了制造过程。这种生产流程的简化不仅降低了能源消耗,而且节省了成本,使产品在不损害环境的情况下具有经济可行性。

该产品在可持续性方面的一个关键要素是使用铝罐。铝的可回收性确保该包装可以一直被重复使用,这与公司的可持续发展目标完全一致。

2024-6 号罐 360 度旋转视频二维码

编号:2024-7

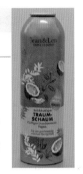

英文介绍

Can No. 7: Jean & Len "Traumschaum" Shower Foam

Marketed Can

Description: With the aerosol can for Jean & Len's shower foam, the manufacturer aimes to demonstrate its expertise in the field of aluminium forming and printing techniques. The product is available in two different fragrances, with the printing evoking expectations of the respective scent. The print image of the "argan oil and fig" shower foam, with its various green leaves in combination with fruits and flowers, is reminiscent of an oriental atmosphere. The main scents of the second variant, oat milk and coconut oil, are also taken up in the illustrative artwork and interpreted with predominantly white and blue tones. Both print versions are realized with metallic background colours applied to a white base coat.

The cans are printed inline. In order to achieve an optimal printing result, the printing colours are well combined and precisely printed. This allows the filigree illustrations to be realised perfectly. The gloss effect is achieved with a colourless topcoat. The cans impress with an extraordinary artwork that helps them stand out on the shop shelf.

中文介绍

7 号罐:

已上市罐

产品说明:

这款为 Jean & Len 公司设计的淋浴泡沫气雾罐展示了制造商在铝成型和印刷技术领域的专业能力。该产品有两种不同的香型,通过不同的印刷图案唤起人们对不同香型的期望。"摩洛哥坚果油和无花果"淋浴泡沫的印刷图案中,有各种绿叶,还有水果和花朵,营造出东方氛围。第二种香型是燕麦牛奶和椰子油,主要香味也在插图设计中得到体现,并主要采用白色和蓝色色调进行诠释。两个印刷版本都是在白色底涂层上应用了金属背景色来实现的。

罐体是在生产线上直接印刷的。为了达到最佳的印刷效果,印刷颜色经过精心搭配并精准印刷,从而可以完美地实现精细的插图效果。光泽效果则是通过一层透明光油实现的。这些罐子以其非凡的艺术设计给人留下深刻印象,使它们在商店货架上脱颖而出。

2024-7号罐360度旋转视频二维码

编号：2024-8

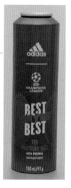

英 文 介 绍

Can No. 8: Adidas Deodorant—UEFA Champions League Edition
Sustainability Can

Description: This deodorant project is a partnership between Adidas and the UEFA Champions League. The artwork for the packaging is created with the global team of the can manufacturer in partnership with Adidas and replicated in all world markets.

The cans technical challenges and sustainability credits are noteworthy. The design highlights fine detailed "fingerprints" on the front of the can, in pink, with the fusion of the background in blue. To achieve this, the manufacturer developed two special blues so that when one was superimposed over the other. There is no visual marking, but rather a smooth passage. To ensure the elements stand out against the background and achieve the desired result, the team developes special inks, bringing more shine and prominence to the elements.

The 45 mm×148 mm aerosol can with flat shoulder is developed using a proprietary advanced aluminum alloy containing up to 25% recycled content and produced through an innovative process where aluminum is used in the liquid phase, removing the need to melt ingots as in the traditional process. It is produced utilizing renewable energy, thus ensuring lower carbon emissions rates. Additionally, the internal varnish used is reduced by almost 50%, contributing to a smaller footprint in greenhouse gas emissions.

中 文 介 绍

8号罐：

可持续发展罐

产品说明：

此款香体剂项目是阿迪达斯与欧洲冠军联赛的合作成果。包装艺术设计是由制罐商的全球团队与阿迪达斯合作完成的，并在全球市场推广。

罐子的技术挑战和可持续性发展成就值得特别关注。该设计在罐子正面突出显示了精细的粉红色"指纹"，与蓝色背景相融合。为了达到这一效果，制造商开发了两种特殊的蓝色，以便将一种蓝色叠印在另一种蓝色上。这种设计不但没有视觉上的不协调，而是呈现平滑的过渡。为了确保图案元素在背景中突出显示并达到预期的效果，团队开发了特殊的油墨，增加了光泽度和视觉冲击力。

这款 45 mm×148 mm 圆肩气雾罐使用了专有的先进铝合金,其中含有高达 25% 的回收成分,并通过创新工艺生产,其中铝在液态下使用,避免了传统工艺中熔化铸锭的过程。这种方法利用了可再生能源,从而确保了较低的碳排放量。此外,使用的内部涂层减少了近 50%,确保该罐在温室气体排放中具有更低的碳足迹。

2024-8 号罐 360 度旋转视频二维码

编号:2024-9

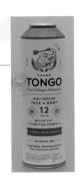

英文介绍

Can No. 9: The Grand Tongo—Town & Jungle Protection

Marketed Can

Description: The brand's commitment to sustainability is evident in its use of sustainably produced aluminum cans, a choice that aligns with the growing consumer demand for eco-friendly packaging solutions.

The 50 mm×165 mm flat shoulder aluminum aerosol can is a great example of technical innovation, reflecting the brand's commitment to excellence and sustainability. The can's design is a result of meticulous research and development, focusing on user-friendliness and environmental impact. One of the most notable features is the use of aluminum, which provides a lightweight and durable container and ensures that the can is recyclable, reducing the product's carbon footprint.

From a technical prespective, the Grand Tongo can has incorporated a bag-on-valve system that allows for a fine mist spray, delivering the repellent effectively and efficiently. This system minimizes waste and ensures that each application is consistent, enhancing the user experience. The can's design also includes a twist-lock cap that prevents accidental discharge, making it safe for transport and storage.

中文介绍

9 号罐:

已上市罐

产品说明:

该品牌对可持续发展的承诺体现在其使用可持续回收利用的铝罐上,这种选择与消费者对环保包装解决方案日益增长的需求相一致。

50 mm×165 mm 圆肩铝气雾罐是技术创新的一个很好的例子,反映了该品牌对卓越和可持续发展的承诺。罐体的创新设计是精心研究和开发的结果,注重用户友好性和环境影响。最显著的特点之一是使用铝材料,它提供了一个轻便又耐用的容器,并确保罐子是可回收的,从而减少了产品的碳足迹。

　　从技术角度来看,Grand Tongo 气雾罐采用了一个阀袋系统,可有效地喷出细腻的喷雾。该系统最大限度地减少了浪费,并确保每次使用时效果一致,从而提升了用户体验。罐体设计还包括一个扭转锁定盖,防止意外喷射,使其在运输和储存时更加安全。

2024-9 号罐 360 度旋转视频二维码

二、2023 年国际铝气雾罐竞赛参赛罐

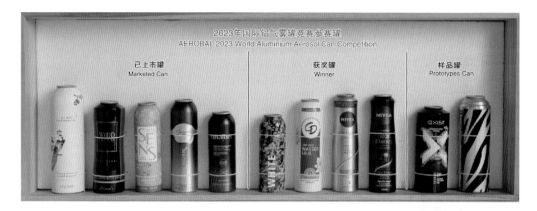

产品编号从左至右分别是：1,3,4,6,2,8,10,11,5,9,7

编号：2023-1

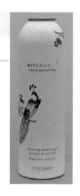

英文介绍

Can No. 1: RITUALS AMSTERDAM COLLECTION Foaming Shower Gel
Marketed Can

Description: A monobloc aerosol can, made of 100% recycled aluminium (100% post consumer recycled), offers a light weight due to the ironing process. This product has been created by RITUALS cosmetic trade in an exclusive partnership with RIJKS Museum in Amsterdam. The design presents a super matt finish with precious "SPOTS of LIGHT" given by golden hot foil stamping. The can maker is certified by an accredited indipendent body, in collaboration with its selected aluminium slugs' suppliers (i. e. the Chain of Custody) to guarantee the origin and quality of the post consumer recycled aluminium.

中文介绍

1 号罐：

已上市罐

产品说明：

　　一款单片铝质气雾罐由 100% 再生铝（100% 消费后再回收）制成，并通过拉伸工艺使其重量更轻。该产品由 RITUALS 化妆品交易所与阿姆斯特丹 RIJKS 博物馆独家合作推出。该设计采用了超哑光的饰面以及金色烫金工艺，呈现了珍贵的"光之亮点"。该铝罐制造商获得了权威的独立机构认证，并与其选定的铝合金供应商（如产销监管链）合作，确保回收再利用铝的来源和质量。

2023-1 号罐 360 度旋转视频二维码

编号:2023-2

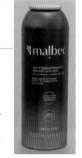

英 文 介 绍

Can No. 2: Malbec X

Marketed Can

Description: Malbec X is created with the aim of raising the level of sensuality for the male gender, meeting the desires of the consumer. Its intense sensual fragrance instills confidence without demands so he can enjoy every moment of conquest. The aerosol format is chosen due to its high level of performance within perfuming, leaving the scent on the body for much longer.

The can incorporates three gradient tones: brown, red and orange. The biggest challenge to the technical aspects of incorporating the design onto the can is keeping all three tones visible. One tone can not cover the other. Covering the smallest of areas in the design, the orange tone is the most challenging bringing forth innovation. To successfully apply the orange a roller is developed by the team allowing the paint to be transferred to the can within a space of 27 mm without contaminating the red tone.

Adding to the print complexity, all actions concerning design and structure of the can focus on sustainably. The can has up to 25% PCR. For this project, all the design is revisited and redesigned in order to reach a high level of sustainability gains. Compared with the previous version, it is possible to reduce around 20% of weight, resulting in approximately a 30% reduction in CO_2 emissions, thereby avoiding consumption more than 100 t of aluminium.

中 文 介 绍

2 号罐:

已上市罐

产品说明:

Malbec X 的诞生旨在提升男性的性感魅力、满足消费者的愿望。它浓郁的感性香味能给人无以伦比的自信,可以让他享受征服的每一刻。选择气雾剂形式是因为它在留香方面的优异表现,可以使香味在身体上停留更久。

该罐结合三种渐变色调:棕色、红色和橙色。将表面的设计融入罐子的最大技术挑战是保持三种色调都清晰可见,一种色调不能覆盖另一种色调。在设计中橙色覆盖最小的区域,是最具挑战性的创新。为了成功地涂上橙色,该团队开发了一种滚涂技术,可以将橙色精准应用于

27 mm 的区域上,而不会污染红色色调。

所有关于罐子的设计和结构的方案都集中在可持续上,从而增加了印刷的复杂性。该罐含有高达25%的再生材料,因此所有设计都被重新审视和改造,以实现可持续性的提升。与以前的版本相比,它可以减少约20%的重量,降低约30%的二氧化碳排放,避免消耗超过100吨的铝材。

2023-2 号罐 360 度旋转视频二维码

编号:2023-3

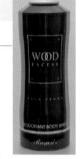

英文介绍

Can No. 3: Rasasi Perfumes Industries Can

Marketed Can

Description: Rasasi Perfumes Industries is a company from the United Arab Emirates founded in 1979. Over the past decades, Rasasi has developed perfumes that are intended to embody the image of quality, luxury and elegance worldwide. The breakthrough in the western world comes with the famous Blue Lady brand. Today, Rasasi is Dubai's largest company in the perfume industry with a global focus and vision. This sophisticated vision is perfectly reflected in the aluminium aerosol cans for the Rasasi deodorant body sprays for men and women produced by the company: premium impression at first sight, high quality material in a breathtaking design, luxury in a perfect staging, artistically inspired by women's trends and fashion. You will feel the quality, sustainability and innovative touches when you hold this can. The artful printing technique gives a new dimension to the customer's brand and equip these really beautiful cans with a personality. From the glamorous overall impression to the smallest detail, filigree lines and patterns give the cans an exquisite touch.

中文介绍

3 号罐:

已上市罐

产品说明:

Rasasi 香水公司来自阿拉伯联合酋长国,成立于1979 年。在过去的几十年里,Rasasi 开发了旨在体现高品质、奢华和优雅形象的香水。西方世界对香水的突破来自著名的 Blue Lady 品牌。如今,Rasasi 是迪拜香水行业最大的具有全球视野的公司。精妙的视觉效果完美地体现在男女 Rasasi 香体剂的铝气雾罐上:第一眼就给人以高端的印象、具有创新的高品质材料、呈现出完美的奢华、艺术灵感来自女性潮流和时尚。当你手持这个罐子时,你会感受到质量、可持续性和创新的细节。巧妙的印刷技术为客户的品牌提供了一个新的维度,使这些极为美丽的罐子拥有了独特的个性。从华丽的整体印象到最细微之处,精细的线条和图案赋予罐体精致的触感。

2023-3 号罐 360 度旋转视频二维码

编号:**2023-4**

英文介绍

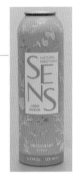

Can No. 4: The Sens Deodorant Spray Can

Marketed Can

Description: The Sens Deodorant Spray by Fragancias Cannon is an innovative and exciting addition to the local deodorant market. Fragancias Cannon, a renowned fragrance company, is launching their Sens brand for the first time in a deodorant applicator, featuring eye-catching and unique artworks inspired by their Sens eau de toilette range, which sets it apart from other products in the market. The artworks are directly printed in bright, vivid colors on aluminum bottles that contain up to 10% recycled content.

中文介绍

4 号罐:

已上市罐

产品说明:

　　由 Fragancias Cannon 推出的 Sens 香体喷雾剂是当地香体剂市场的一款具有创新且令人兴奋的产品。著名香水公司 Fragancias Cannon 首次在香体剂中推出了 Sens 品牌,其设计灵感来自 Sens 淡香水系列,这些引人注目且独特的产品,使其在市场上脱颖而出。艺术作品直接以明亮、生动的颜色被印刷在含有 10% 可回收成分的铝罐上。

2023-4 号罐 360 度旋转视频二维码

编号:2023-5

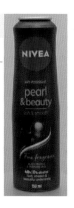

英文介绍

Can No. 5: Pearl & Beauty

Marketed Can

Description: The can's design is truly outstanding, featuring with an eye-catching colour scheme. The dark aubergine colour is translucent and the extremely fine brushing of the aluminium shines through and gives the whole can a sparkling effect. The pearl is the centerpiece of the design, and it is superbly printed displaying the finest gradients.

For these gradients the copy dot technique is used. This artwork technique is used here to create the sparkling and shining of the pearl.

The challenge lies in applying the right amount of ink on a dark background while ensuring there is no contamination of the lighter colour by the darker one as the details of the design printed would not be visible. This technique is used to highlight design elements. As the centerpiece shows, the copy dot artwork technique is mastered superbly.

中文介绍

5号罐:

已上市罐

产品说明:

这款罐体的设计非常出色,它采用了吸引眼球的色彩方案。深紫红色是半透明的,非常精细地刷涂在铝罐上,使整个罐体呈现出一个闪闪发光的效果。珍珠是设计的核心,它印刷精美,显示出微妙的渐变效果。

为了实现渐变效果,使用复制点技术,使得珍珠闪闪发光。其挑战在于在深色背景上应用适量的油墨,并确保较浅的颜色不会受到较深颜色的污染,否则设计细节将无法呈现。这种技术适合突出设计元素。正如设计核心的珍珠那样,复制点技术掌握得非常好。

2023-5号罐360度旋转视频二维码

编号:2023-6

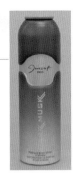

英文介绍

Can No. 6: 45 mm×150 mm Emboss for Jacsaf

Marketed Can

Description: Jacsaf is a new brand of Elysee Kish perfumery company which is very well known in Iran with a wide range of high-quality perfume and personal care products. For their premium perfumed body spray project, Elysee Kish company needs an innovative aluminium can solution to their new body spray projects.

After a long study on the aluminium can type, the customer makes a decision on the innovative technology called "360° Embossed Shaping with Oriented Printing". The type of the embossed shape is very unique and the brand "JACSAF" has been highlighted on the embossed part of the aerosol can.

中文介绍

6 号罐:

已上市罐

产品说明:

Jacsaf 是 Elysee Kish 香水公司的一个新品牌,该公司在伊朗非常有名,拥有各种高品质的香水和个人护理产品。对于他们全新的身体喷雾项目,Elysee Kish 公司需要一种创新的铝罐解决方案。

经过对铝罐类型的长期研究,客户决定采用名为"360°浮雕成型与定向印刷"的创新技术。气雾剂罐上的浮雕形状非常独特,在气雾剂罐的浮雕部分其中突出显示了"JACSAF"商标。

2023-6 号罐 360 度旋转视频二维码

编号:2023-7

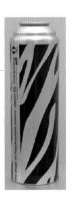

英文介绍

Can No. 7: Rainbow Can

Prototypes Can

Description: The can is printed in combination of classic UV silkscreen printing (black) and an additional silkscreen print (polychromatic ink) that is thermically cured. To combine both curing systems on one can is a challenge. UV is fast drying whereas the thermically cured ink needs more time for curing. To make sure the design is pin sharp, the rheology of both inks—especially the polychromatic ink—has to be taken into account. The perfect colour application is essential in order to display the rainbow effect. Less ink means little to no effect, the use of too much ink would end up in a blurry design.

The effect of the polychromatic ink adapts to the ambient light and gives the can a unique and luxurious design. The polychromatic ink opens a whole new colour cosmos as the rainbow effect—especially in sun light—literally explodes and displays a multitude of colours. Like the multitude of colours, brands have—with this printing technique—a multitude of exciting design options.

中文介绍

7号罐:

样品罐

产品说明:

该罐是由经典的紫外线固化的丝网印刷(黑色)和热固化的额外丝网印刷(多色油墨)相结合的方式进行印刷的。将两种固化系统结合在一个罐子上是一个挑战。紫外线固化得快,而热固化则需要更长的时间。为了确保设计的精致,两种油墨的流变性——尤其是多色油墨——必须考虑在内。为了显示彩虹般效果,完美的色彩应用是必不可少的。油墨越少,效果就越弱,油墨越多,设计就越模糊。

多色油墨的效果随着光线的变化而变化,使罐体具有独特而奢华的设计感。多色油墨开启了一个全新的色彩世界,彩虹效应——尤其是在阳光下——能够完美地曝光和呈现出多种颜色。就像多种色彩一样,使用这种印刷技术可以设计出多种令人兴奋的商标图案。

2023-7号罐360度旋转视频二维码

编号:2023-8

英文介绍

Can No. 8: The Smart Sustainable Aerosol Can

Prototypes Can

Description: The smart sustainable aerosol can is a moduct of cooperation, manufactured with our partner, the Italian coating supplier SalchiMetalcoatSrl. This innovative can unites sustainability and functionality without compromising on performance, safety and durability.

The can body is manufactured from 100% post-consumer-recycled aluminium, which is originating from used beverage can scrap with no addition of virgin or post-industrial-recycled material.

The patented Nucan-PCR alloy has been awarded DIN EN ISO 14021 certification, attesting transparency and traceability of the value chain from the used drink can to the finished Nucan-PCR can. This can-to-can upcycling concept saves 96% of CO_2. The clear and white basecoat as well as the clear overprint varnish applied to the cans are bio-based polyester coatings from Sachi's BIOMOCO line. The name stands for biosustainable modern coatings and summarizes the company's coating portfolio made from castor oil and waste cooking oil, which partly replace traditional fossil-based materials. The coatings convince with excellent mechanic properties, very good elasticity, low VOC content and they are of course hot water bath resistant. The bio-content on solid is more than 40%.

Finally, also the inner lining chosen is of the latest generation. It is a non-BPA epoxy gold lacquer, combining the excellent compatibility properties of EP coatings with the advantage of a bisphenol A-free lacquer solution.

中文介绍

8 号罐:

样品罐

产品说明:

　　智能可持续气雾罐是与我们的合作伙伴意大利涂料供应商 SalchiMetalcoatSrl 合作生产的。这种创新可以将可持续性和功能性结合起来,而不会影响性能、安全性和耐用性。

　　罐身 100% 由消费后回收铝制成,这种铝来自用过的饮料罐废料,不添加原生或工业后回收材料。专利技术 Nucan-PCR 合金已获得欧盟 ISO 14021 认证,证明了从废旧饮料罐到 Nucan-PCR 成品罐的价值链的透明度和可追溯性。这种罐到罐的升级循环概念可以减少 96% 的二氧化碳排放。白色透明的底涂层以及适用于罐子的透明光油来自 Sachi 的 BIOMOCO 生产线的生物基聚酯涂料。该名称代表生物可持续现代涂料,概括了该公司由蓖麻油和废弃食用油制成的涂料组合,部分取代了传统的化石材料。该涂料具有优异的机械性能、良好的弹性、低含量的有机化合物挥发性,以及耐热水浴处理。固体中的生物基含量大于 40%。

　　最后,气雾罐也选择了最新一代的内部涂层。它是一种不含双酚 A 的环氧金色内涂,结合了环氧树脂涂料的优异相容性和不含双酚 A 涂层的优点。

2023-8 号罐 360 度旋转视频二维码

编号:2023-9

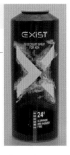

英文介绍

Can No. 9: 53 mm×140 mm Flat for EXIST Sailor & Energy Prototypes Can

Description: These cans have been printed with neon pantone colours which are super visible and shiny in the dark under UV led light. Thanks to the printing technique, the company has proved its printing quality even with neon colours as a concept product.

中文介绍

9 号罐:

样品罐

产品说明:

这些罐体使用了荧光潘通色进行印刷,在紫外灯照射下,它们在黑暗中非常显眼,且闪闪发光。得益于这项印刷技术,该公司展示了即使在使用荧光色时,其印刷质量仍能达到高标准,作为概念产品非常出色。

2023-9 号罐 360 度旋转视频二维码

编号:2023-10

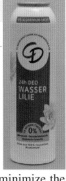

英文介绍

Can No. 10: Lornamead's CD Deodorants

Sustainability Can

Description: These 150 mL aerosol cans (45 mm×150 mm) for Lornamead's CD deodorants are made from 17% lighter slugs and consist of an alloy with 100% post-consumer recycled PCR aluminium and 0. 3% virgin manganese. As the most sustainable material is the one that is not used at all, the first goal of this packaging is to minimize the material use while meeting the stability requirements of a deodorant aerosol can. The second objective of the project is to cut the can's carbon footprint via post-consumer recycled aluminium. This innovative can saves 296. 5 t CO_2 per million cans.

Unlike most PCR slugs, the slugs used by our company are produced directly from molten aluminium scrap without an energy-consuming second melting process. Due to this, the results of our life cycle assessments show that PCR slugs are characterized by a very low carbon footprint of 1. 1 kg CO_2e/kg. This allows saving of 92% compared to our virgin slugs (13. 1 kg CO_2e/kg) and probably even more when compared to other slugs available on the market. Thus, in total, 296.5 t CO_2 can be saved per million cans. Additionally, the reduced weight also saves transport emissions.

The supply chain is traceable in accordance with ISO 22095:2020. High security of supply is ensured by high material availability and secured quantities. The 150 mL CD deodorant aerosol cans are an excellent combination of material reduction and recyclate use.

中 文 介 绍

10 号罐:

可持续发展罐

产品说明:

Lornamead 公司的 150 mL CD 香体剂气雾罐(45 mm×150 mm)由 17% 的较轻铝片制成,包含 100% 消费后回收铝和 0.3% 的原生锰制成的合金。由于最可持续的材料是根本不消耗的材料,这种包装的首要目标是尽量减少材料的使用,同时满足香体剂气雾罐的稳定性要求;第二个目标是通过使用消费后回收铝来减少罐体的碳足迹。通过这种创新,每百万罐可减少 296.5 t 二氧化碳排放。

与大多数消费后回收铝不同,Lornamead 公司使用的铝片直接从熔融铝废料中生产,没有二次熔化过程的能源消耗。因此,生命周期评估结果显示,消费后回收的铝片碳足迹非常低,为 1.1 kg CO_2e/kg。与使用原始铝片(13.1 kg CO_2e/kg)生产相比,可以节省 92% 的碳排放,与市场上的其他铝片相比,甚至可能更多。这样,每百万罐可减少 296.5 t 二氧化碳排放。此外,罐体重量的减轻也减少了运输过程中产生的排放。

该产品的供应链可根据 ISO 22095:2020 进行追溯。材料的高度可用性和数量的可保障性确保了供应的高度安全性。这款 150 mL 的 CD 香体剂气雾罐是减少原料使用和可回收材料利用的绝佳组合。

2023-10 号罐 360 度旋转视频二维码

编号:**2023-11**

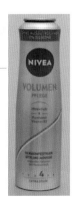

英 文 介 绍

Can No.11: Nivea Volumen Pflege

Sustainability Can

Description: This can is unique and proofs that a closed loop concept is feasible for aluminium monobloc cans, too. In general, the patented alloy Neucan 3.1 combines advantages of significant weight reduction and a possible inclusion of real PCR. This can is made with 50% real PCR inclusion and the decoration is printed with natural colours. The holistic approach is optimized by using pure organic inks beside all other well-known advantages of this first time ever natural ink.

Details of distinction: The novelty is the unique way of the recycling process of the material used as real PCR in this can! Not only recycled material is used, but the company is also concerned where it comes from and how the recycled material is processed to be brought back into the life cycle.

中文介绍

11 号罐:

可持续发展罐

产品说明:

这款罐子独具特色,也证明铝制气雾罐作为一个封闭循环概念是可行的。总的来说,专利 Neucan 3.1 合金技术结合了显著减轻重量和真正消费后回收的优点。这种罐体含有 50% 的消费后回收原料,其表面印刷使用天然颜料。除了所有其他众所周知的优势外,这是有史以来第一次优化使用纯有机天然油墨。

区别的细节:创新之处在于使用材料作为真实 PCR(消费后回收材料)的独特回收过程。该公司不仅使用回收材料,还关注这些材料的来源以及如何处理回收材料使其重新进入生命周期。

2023-11 号罐 360 度旋转视频二维码

三、2022 年国际铝气雾罐竞赛参赛罐

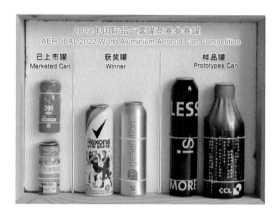

产品编号从左至右分别是:5,5-1,1,4,2,3

编号:2022-1

英 文 介 绍

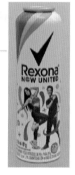

Can No. 1: Rexona Now United

Marketed Can

Description: As the official dance partner of Now United, Rexona's graphics showcase bright vivid colors, and express the values of the group, instilling confidence that the product provides the protection the consumer needs to move as they want!

The design reflects the fans' desire to see the members of Now United on the bottle. The challenging design requires a significant level of hands-on work to ensure the faces are of the highest quality in printing all while maintaining Rexona brand positioning, group approval, and technical feasibility.

The visuals celebrate the group members, movement, and dance. Rich in details, their faces and bodies are overlaid with colors and graphics, a challenging technical aspect of the design that required Trivium to capture all the nuances of expressions using 8-color dry-offset technology.

The aluminum packaging is launched using an advanced alloy developed by the producer that contains recycled content, enabling it's lightweight and contributing to reduced consumption of aluminum with sustainable impacts on the overall supply chain.

In addition, the deodorant can's design includes a QR Code, that connects consumers with a new exclusive dance content hub, a new media platform that allows for the intrinsic connection between brand, product and content.

中文介绍

1号罐：

已上市罐

产品说明：

作为 Now United 官方舞蹈合作伙伴，Rexona 的图形展示了明亮生动的色彩，并表达了该群体的价值观，增强了消费者对产品提供保需保护的信心！

这种设计反映了粉丝们希望看到 Now United 成员出现在瓶子上的愿望。这项具有挑战性的设计需要大量的手工工作，确保表面达到最高的印刷质量，同时保持 Rexona 品牌的定位、集团认可和技术可行性。

视觉效果呈现了团队成员及其动作和舞蹈。设计细节丰富，他们的脸和身体上都有丰富的颜色和图形，这是设计中一个具有挑战性的技术，要求 Trivium 使用 8 色干式胶印技术捕捉所有表情的细微差别。

铝包装采用了由生产商开发的一种含有回收成分的先进合金，其重量轻，有助于减少铝的消耗，并对整个供应链产生可持续的影响。

此外，香体剂罐的设计包括一个二维码，将消费者与一个新的独家舞蹈内容中心联系起来，这是一个新媒体平台，可以在品牌、产品和内容之间建立内在联系。

2022-1 号罐 360 度旋转视频二维码

编号：2022-2

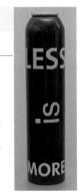

英文介绍

Can No. 2: Less is More

Prototypes Can

Description: This can shows the latest development in overvarnish. An overvarnish was not thought possible. So far standard (not water-based) overvarnishes are based on Polyester, which originates from mineral oil. Water-based overvarnish has 10% conventional solvents. This overvarnish has little amount of biodegradable solvents!

This overvarnish has no fossil carbon (no mineral oil, no ingredients that are based on mineral oil), no use of heavy metal, no labelling needed, not hazardous, no odour, no need of after burning, and the used ingredients are biodegradable.

The using and processing of mineral oil leaves a high carbon foot print. With the use of pure overvarnish the carbon footprint has been significantly lowered. Finally an ecological friendly overvarnish for aluminium cans.

The manufacturer has worked with natural ink (the design is printed with natural ink) and it is logic to go to the next step and develop with the supplier of said ink a whole new overvarnish.

中 文 介 绍

2 号罐：

样品罐

产品说明：

这个罐子展示了光油的最新发展。这种光油以前被认为是无法实现的。到目前为止,标准的(非水基的)光油是基于聚酯的,它来源于矿物油。水性光油中含有10%的常规溶剂。这种光油仅含有少量可生物降解的溶剂!

这种光油不含化石碳(不含矿物油,不含矿物油成分)、不含重金属、不需要标签、无危险物质、没有气味、不需要二次燃烧、使用的成分均可生物降解。

矿物油的使用和生产会产生较高的碳足迹,而使用纯光油后,碳足迹显著降低,由此产生了生态友好型的光油铝罐。

制造商使用了天然油墨(设计就是用天然油墨印刷的),下一步是与油墨供应商一起开发一种全新的光油。

2022-2 号罐 360 度旋转视频二维码

编号：2022-3

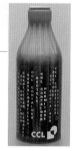

英 文 介 绍

Can No. 3: Self-promotional Aerosol Container

Prototypes Can

Description: For the 2022 Aerobal World Aluminum Aerosol Can Award, the producer is pleased to submit a self-promotional aerosol container that embodies multiple distinctive attributes.

Unique shaping—the flute form design provides a striking visual effect along with a vertical grip feature created to enhance the application experience.

Eye-catching graphics—the background fade from green to black over a clear basecoat provides a great look, but also a challenge. The producer incorporates split well ink technologies to deliver smooth color transition without the pixelated look of a half tone screen. In addition to a color fade, the text is depleted or starved to also fade into the fluted form element.

Sustainability message—the color combination and art is created to aid in the promotion of environmental sustainability and to highlight the role aluminum recycling plays within. Sustainability is absolutely key within our company, our industry, our customers, retailers and consumers.

中文介绍

3 号罐：

样品罐

产品说明：

对于 2022 年世界铝气雾罐奖，生产商很高兴提交一款具有多种防尘特性的带有自我宣传的气雾剂容器。

独特的形状——长笛形式的设计提供了引人注目的视觉效果，以及垂直握持功能，以提高应用体验。

引人注目的图案——背景在一个透明底涂层上从绿色到黑色，呈现出极佳的外观，同时也带来了挑战。生产商采用了分体式油墨技术，实现了颜色的平滑过渡，避免了半色调显示的像素化效果。除了颜色渐变，文字也逐渐消失，与笛形元素完美融合。

可持续性的信息——色彩组合和艺术设计有助于促进环境的可持续性，并突出铝回收在其中所起的作用。可持续性绝对是我们公司、行业、客户、零售商和消费者们的核心理念。

2022-3 号罐 360 度旋转视频二维码

编号：2022-4

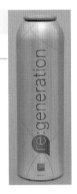

英文介绍

Can No. 4: re: generation

Prototypes Can

Description: This year the producer entered a new era of sustainable packaging grounded in the mission to re-define aluminum aerosol packaging. By re-imagining, re-thinking, re-building, and re-placing the current landscape of aerosol packaging, Ball has achieved a 50% reduction in carbon footprint (compared to a standard aluminum aerosol can) and launched its most sustainable aerosol can to date.

The re: gen can demonstrates what can be achieved when ReAl® (Ball's proprietary and pate-hted alloy composition, 50% recycled content) and low-carbon primary aluminum sourced from renewable energy sources like hydroelectric power (which generates 75% less CO_2e compared to global average for aluminum production) are combined. The cans produced are up to 30% lighter, compared to a standard aluminum aerosol cans, while retaining strength, structure, and preserving package integrity requirements.

The impact of lightweighting is significant: less weight and less raw material means significantly less energy used in production and transportation. Ball is committed to providing globally impactful solutions and the re: gen cans, available on a global scale, are no exception.

Ball continues to take a holistic approach to identify opportunities throughout the product life-cycle and in doing so, delivers innovative packaging solutions that will help people live more sustainably and improve the health of the planet. And this is only the beginning.

中文介绍

4号罐：

样品罐

产品说明：

今年生产商迈入了可持续包装的新时代,其使命是重新定义铝气雾剂包装。通过重新构想、重新思考、重新构建和替换现有的气雾剂包装,Ball 公司已经实现了碳足迹减少 50%(与标准铝制气雾剂罐相比),并推出了迄今为止最具可持续性的气雾剂罐。

re:gen 罐展示了 ReAl 专利(Ball 公司独有的合金成分、50%的可回收成分)和来自水力发电等可再生能源的低碳原铝(与全球铝生产平均水平相比,其产生的二氧化碳排放量减少了75%)相结合所能取得的成就。与标准铝气雾罐相比,Ball 公司生产的罐体重量减轻了 30%,同时保持了强度、结构和包装完整性。

轻量化的影响是显著的:更轻的重量和更少的原材料意味着在生产和运输中使用的能源大大减少。Ball 公司致力于提供具有全球影响力的解决方案,在全球范围内提供循环回收罐。

Ball 公司继续采取整体性方法,在整个产品生命周期中寻找机会,并在此过程中提供创新的包装解决方案,帮助人们更可持续地生活,改善地球的健康。而这仅仅是个开始。

2022-4 号罐 360 度旋转视频二维码

编号：2022-5

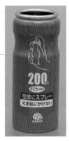

英文介绍

Can No. 5: Aerosol Can 200

Marketed Can

Description: The aerosol can with a body is curved for easy gripping and spraying.

中文介绍

5号罐：

已上市罐

产品说明：

这款气雾剂罐的罐身设计为弧形,便于抓握和喷洒。

2022-5 号罐 360 度旋转视频二维码

编号: **2022-5-1**

英文介绍

Can No. 5-1: Aerosol Can 120

Marketed Can

Description: The aerosol cans with a body is curved for easy gripping and spraying.

中文介绍

5-1 号罐：

已上市罐

产品说明：

　　这款气雾剂罐的罐身设计为弧形，便于抓握和喷洒。

2022-5-1 号罐 360 度旋转视频二维码

四、2021年国际铝气雾罐竞赛参赛罐

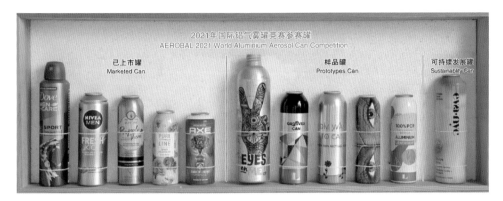

产品编号从左至右分别是：11,7,13,3,12,14,4,9,8,5,2

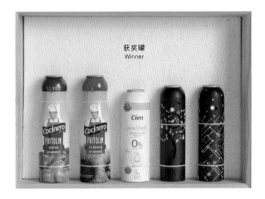

产品编号从左至右分别是：1,1-1,6,10,10-1

编号：2021-1

英文介绍

Can No.1: Cocinero Fritolim Oliva and Clasico

Marketed Can

Description: Cocinero Fritolim Oliva is an edible oil spray focused on bringing quality and portion control to health-minded consumers. Consumers looking to reduce their calories can control their intake as the spray allows the user control over the spread of the oil resulting in less oil use and thus fewer calories are consumed.

Cocinero oils come in three varieties: Clasico, Oliva, and Butter. Through exemplary design, each showcases the brand's iconic hallmark, a distinguished-looking man in his apron and chef hat, smiling back at the user. Achieving the iconic look is of utmost importance in the new packaging.

To achieve it in conjunction with the shape of the can is a challenge that required attention to detail and precision, distorting the face of the man in pre-production graphics so when applied in production it appeared crisp, clean, and proportional despite the shape of the aerosol can.

The cans reflect healthy choices, beauty, and sustainability. A key factor in this success is the use of sustainable materials that contribute to better products for the Argentina market. Cocinero oils are produced using recycled aluminum content. This infinitely recyclable packaging reflects the company's mission to provide more valuable, healthy, and accessible products to consumers.

中 文 介 绍

1 号罐：

已上市罐

产品说明：

　　Cocinero Friitolim Oliva 是一款食用油喷雾罐,专注于为注重健康的消费者对食用油的质量和用量的控制。希望减少卡路里的消费者可以控制食用油的摄入量,因为喷雾允许用户控制油的释放量,减少油的使用,从而减少摄入的卡路里。

　　Cocinero 油有三种：Clasico、Oliva 和 Butter。通过堪称典范的设计,每一款都展示了该品牌的标志性图案：一个穿着围裙、戴着厨师帽、看起来很尊贵的微笑着的男子。在新包装中,使用标志性的外观是很重要的。将图案与罐子的形状结合起来是一个挑战,需要注意细节和精度,需要在前期设计图形时对人物的面部进行精确调整,才能在实际生产应用时仍能保持图像的清晰、干净和比例协调。

　　这些罐子反映了人们对健康的选择、对美的追求和可持续性。成功的关键因素是使用可持续材料,这有助于为阿根廷市场提供更好的产品。Cocinero 食用油喷雾罐是用回收铝生产的。这种可无限循环利用的包装反映了公司致力于为消费者提供更有价值、更健康、更容易获取产品的使命。

2021-1 号罐 360 度旋转视频二维码

编号：2021-1-1

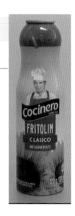

英 文 介 绍

Can No. 1-1: Cocinero Fritolim Oliva and Clasico

Marketed Can

Description: Cocinero Fritolim Oliva is an edible oil spray focused on bringing quality and portion control to health-minded consumers. Consumers looking to reduce their calories can control their intake as the spray allows the user control over the spread of the oil resulting in less oil use and thus fewer calories are consumed.

Cocinero oils come in three varieties: Clasico, Oliva, and Butter. Through exemplary design, each showcases the brand's iconic hallmark, a distinguished-looking man in his apron and chef hat, smiling back at the user. Achieving the iconic look is of utmost importance in the new packaging. To achieve it in conjunction with the shape of the can is a challenge that required attention to detail and precision, distorting the face of the man in pre-production graphics so when applied in production it appeared crisp, clean, and proportional despite the shape of the aerosol can.

The cans reflect healthy choices, beauty, and sustainability. A key factor in this success is the use of sustainable materials that contribute to better products for the Argentina market. Cocinero oils are produced using recycled aluminum content. This infinitely recyclable packaging reflects the company's mission to provide more valuable, healthy, and accessible products to consumers.

中文介绍

1-1 号罐：

已上市罐

产品说明：

Cocinero Fritolim Oliva 是一款食用油喷雾罐，专注于为注重健康的消费者对食用油的质量和用量的控制。希望减少卡路里的消费者可以控制食用油的摄入量，因为喷雾允许用户控制油的释放量，减少油的使用，从而减少摄入的卡路里。

Cocinero 油有三种：Clasico、Oliva 和 Butter。通过堪称典范的设计，每一款都展示了该品牌的标志性图案：一个穿着围裙、戴着厨师帽、看起来很尊贵的微笑着的男子。在新包装中，使用标志性的外观是很重要的。将图案与罐子的形状结合起来是一个挑战，需要注意细节和精度，需要在前期设计图形时对人物的面部进行精确调整，才能在生产应用时保持图像的清晰、干净和比例合适。

这些罐子反映了人们对健康的选择、对美的追求和可持续性。成功的关键因素是使用可持续材料，这有助于为阿根廷市场提供更好的产品。Cocinero 食用油喷雾罐是用回收铝生产的。这种可循环回收利用的包装反映了公司致力于为消费者提供更有价值、更健康、更容易获得产品的使命。

2021-1-1 号罐 360 度旋转视频二维码

编号：2021-2

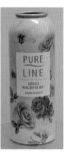

英文介绍

Can No. 2: EVA NYC

Sustainability Can

Description: EVA NYC hair spray(s) features a stylish and bold package design, using colors in an eye-catching and inspiring way. Significant effort goes into creating a more sustainable package for the customer, including using 25% recycled aluminum and decreasing the can weight by nearly 25% over the legacy container.

EVA NYC has become an incredible advocate for aluminum, transitioning its entire hair care product line from plastic to aluminum packaging, all while promoting the benefits of infinitely recyclable aluminum. As a result the company has reported an exponential growth in sales. Customers are thrilled with the new aluminum packaging and its sustainable qualities.

中文介绍

2号罐：

可持续罐

产品说明：

描述：EVA NYC 发胶具有时尚和大胆的包装设计，用了吸引眼球和鼓舞人心的色彩。我们付出了巨大的努力，为客户创造可持续的包装，包括使用 25% 的可回收材料，并将罐体重量比传统罐子减轻近 25%。

EVA NYC 已成为铝包装的积极倡导者，将其整个护发产品线从塑料包装转变为铝包装，同时极力宣传循环可回收铝的好处。因此，该公司的销售额呈指数级增长。客户对新的铝包装及其可持续品质感到非常满意。

2021-2 号罐 360 度旋转视频二维码

编号：2021-3

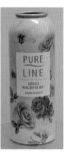

英文介绍

Can No. 3: Pureline

Marketed Can

Description: The producer has been producing aluminum aerosol cans for Unilever for a long while. The spray colognes that are prepared for the Pureline, a brand of Unilever, have taken their place on shelves.

COVID-19 epidemic on again proves that hand hygiene is extremely important. Brands contestes to offer cologne in different concepts and forms, or traditional packaging shapes with recent trends.

The history of cologne in Turkish culture and traditions goes back to old decades. It has been an established and well recognized tradition to offer guests right after settling and before serving tea or coffee. This traditional cologne is usually contained in a glass or plastic bottle from past to present. Instead of the usual bottle packaging, this product is presented in an aerosol cans that could be carried by customers more easily. It is intended to reflect the refreshing feeling of the cologne in the design that produced with 3 different scents such as flower, sea minerals and lime. Designing with simplicity, clear printing, and specified color aim to accommodate only the needs of the end-user.

The artwork has been expressing itself effortlessly, providing necessary instructions to the consumers with its smooth printed high-quality infographics and pitches out excessive designs or innovations.

The producer once again has proven its innovative and flexible approach to fulfill the market demands with a non-traditional way.

中 文 介 绍

3 号罐:

已上市罐

产品说明:

　　该生产商长期以来一直为联合利华生产铝制气雾剂罐,为联合利华旗下的 PURELINE 品牌准备的喷雾香水已经上架。

　　2019 年新型冠状病毒感染疫情再次证明了手部卫生的重要性。品牌商们竞相推出以不同概念和形式的古龙香水,或者采用最新流行的传统包装。

　　古龙香水在土耳其文化和传统中的历史可以追溯到几十年前。通常在客人落座和享用茶或咖啡之前向客人提供古龙水是一项历史悠久且广为人知的传统。这种传统的古龙水通常被装在玻璃或塑料瓶中,从过去到现在都是如此。

　　这款产品没有采用传统的瓶装包装,而是采用了更便于携带的喷雾罐包装。设计中融入了花香、海洋矿物和青柠三种不同的香气,旨在反映古龙水的清新感受。采用简洁的印刷和特定的颜色设计,旨在满足最终用户的需求。

　　艺术作品以简洁的方式表达自己,用其高质量的印刷流畅的图案为消费者提供必要的指导,摒弃了不必要的设计或创新。生产商再次用非传统的方式证明了其创新灵活的理念,以满足市场需求。

2021-3 号罐 360 度旋转视频二维码

编号：2021-4

Can No. 4: Grooved Can

Prototypes Can

Description: The surface of the producer's Grooved Can is not only a visual eye-catcher but also features a tactile experience that clearly differentiates our cans at the point of purchase from traditional cans with smooth surfaces.

Modified pressing tools allow us to create haptic, parallel grooves that can be customized in terms of length, width and positioning. Beside the visual impact, the grooves also provide a "grip zone" for enhanced user convenience.

As the can's surface stays smooth on the inside, applying the inner lacquer is no problem at all and ensures that lacquering process fully meets its protective function. With this technically refined product we've created an entirely new design aesthetic for aerosol cans!

4号罐：

样品罐

产品说明：

该生产商的表面带凹槽纹的罐不仅具有视觉吸引力，而且在触摸体验方面也与传统光滑表面的罐子有明显区别，从而在货架上可以脱颖而出。

经过修改的压模工具使我们能够创建具有触感的平行凹槽，这些凹槽的长度、宽度和位置均可根据需要进行定制。除了视觉效果外，凹槽还为用户提供了一个"抓握区域"，以提高使用的便利性。

由于罐子的内表面光滑，因此在内部涂层不会有任何问题，并确保涂层过程完全能够达到其保护功能。凭借这项技术精湛的产品，我们为气雾罐创造了一种全新的设计美学！

2021-4号罐360度旋转视频二维码

编号:2021-5

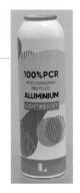

英文介绍

Can No. 5: PCR Aerosol Can

Prototypes Can

Description: At this producer, reduction and using of recycled materials are two of the main drivers for the development of sustainable products. Our new PCR aerosol cans contain over 99% post-consumer recycled aluminum from transparent and traceable sources. The added alloy material increases the hardness of the can creating an additional benefit by making it possible to reduce the wall thickness and use less material. In comparison to conventional aerosol cans made of 99.5% aluminum, the weight savings amount to about 17%.

This aerosol can is sustainable in two ways and thereby enables us to not only save energy, material and CO_2 emissions, but even contribute to a closed material loop—all according to our consistently pursued sustainability strategy of "reduce+replace+recycle".

中文介绍

5号罐:

样品罐

产品说明:

对生产商来说,减少和使用回收材料是可持续产品开发的两个主要驱动因素。我们的新款 PCR 气雾罐含有超过 99% 的回收铝,其来源透明且可追溯。添加的合金材料增加了罐的硬度,并且具有减少壁厚和使用更少材料的优势。与传统的 99.5% 铝制气雾剂罐相比,PCR 气雾罐的重量节省了约 17%。

该款气雾剂罐在两方面都具有可持续性,不仅能够节省能源和材料、减少二氧化碳排放,而且有助于形成一个闭环的材料循环——所有这些都符合我们一贯奉行的"减少+替代+回收"的可持续发展战略。

2021-5 号罐 360 度旋转视频二维码

编号：2021-6

英 文 介 绍

Can No. 6: Cien Deodorant

Sustainability Can

Description: Sustainability is on everyone's agenda but some claims by companies, leave room for interpretation. The manufacturer of this can puts its emphasis on sustainability that can be proven and does not want to participate in greenwashing.

This is the first aluminium aerosol can printed with ecological and sustainable ink. The ink is free of mineral-, palm-, soybean- and cooconut-oil—stops deforestation of the rain forrest. Furthermore no genetically modified organisms are added and the binding agents are completely based on renewable sources. Because of its natural ingredients, this ink is free of labeling.

There are more facts making this deodorant can currently the most sustainable can on the market: patented alloy and due to the alloy light weight (6% less than the predessor can), 25% real PCR inclusion (own closed loop from consumer waste [yellow bin/bag]), natural sustainable ink, water-based overvarnish (less solvents by 60%).

＊Yellow bin/bag collects packaging waste from end consumers for recycling.

中 文 介 绍

6 号罐：

可持续发展罐

产品说明：

可持续发展是每个人的议事日程,但一些公司的声明却存在模糊之处。这家制造商专注于可证实的可持续性,并不希望参与"绿色洗白"行为。

这是第一款使用生态可持续油墨印刷的铝制喷雾罐。这种油墨不含矿物油、棕榈油、大豆油和椰子油,可防止雨林砍伐。此外,未添加转基因生物,粘合剂完全基于可再生资源。由于其天然成分,该油墨无需贴标签。

还有更多事实使这款香体剂罐成为目前市场上最可持续的罐子。专利合金和合金的轻重量使其比前一代罐子轻6%,包含25%的消费后回收材料是从消费者废弃物的黄袋/箱中回收。天然可持续油墨和水基上光油减少溶剂60%。

＊黄袋/箱收集是对消费者的包装废弃物进行回收。

2021-6号罐360度旋转视频二维码

编号：2021-7

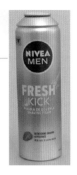

英 文 介 绍

Can No. 7: Nivea Men Fresh Kick

Marketed Can

Description: The decoration of this light weight can (10% less than the former can due to use of alloy) harmonizes perfecty with its content. The material aluminium is used as a masculine design element. The extremely fine brushed aluminium is finished with a semi-matt overvarnish which gives the aluminium and this can a cool and icy look. This iciness is enhanced by the turquois center piece with its extremly fine gradient-resembling an iced window or glass. A perfect example of a combination between material, design and art of printing.

中 文 介 绍

7 号罐：

已上市罐

产品说明：

由于采用了合金材料,这款罐的重量比旧款罐轻了 10%。铝材作为一种表现男性阳刚气质的设计元素,与罐子完美融合。极其精细的磨砂铝表面经过哑光油处理,使铝材罐子呈现出凉爽和冰冷的外观。

这种冰冷感通过对中心部分的蓝色装饰得以增强,其具有极细的渐变效果,仿佛冰冻的窗户或玻璃。这是材料设计与印刷艺术完美结合的典范。

2021-7 号罐 360 度旋转视频二维码

编号：2021-8

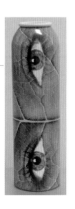

英 文 介 绍

Can No. 8: Most Sustainable Aluminium Monobloc Can in the World

Prototypes Can

Description: This is the ultimate most sustainable aerosol can in the world. This can has every ingredient in terms of sustainability that is available today and can be manufactured industrially:

Alloy with up to 60% real PCR inclusion (closed loop)

Internal powder coating BPA-NI (also partly application)

Decorated with natural ink (The ink is free of mineral-, palm-, soybean- and coconut-oil—no deforestation of rain forrest. No genetically modified organisms are added and the binding agents are completely based on renewable sources. The ink is free of labeling.)

Water based overvarnish (less solvents by 80%)

Light weight, up to 20% lighter

Fully recyclable

This can contains everything there is to manufacture the most sustainable aluminium aerosol monobloc can in the world.

中文介绍

8 号罐：

样品罐

产品说明：

这是世界上最可持续的喷雾罐。该罐包含了目前可用的所有可持续材料,并且可以进行工业化生产。

合金中包含高达 60% 的真正消费后回收材料(闭环)

内部采用无无双酚 A 的粉末涂料(部分应用)

采用天然油墨印刷(油墨不含矿物油、棕榈油、大豆油和椰子油,不会导致雨林砍伐,不含转基因成分,粘合剂完全基于可再生资源。油墨不需贴专门的标签说明)

采用水性上光油(溶剂减少 80%)

重量减轻 20%

完全可回收

该罐包含了制造世界上最可持续的铝制喷雾罐所需的所有材料。

2021-8 号罐 360 度旋转视频二维码

编号：2021-9

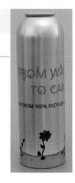

英文介绍

Can No. 9: From Waste to Can

Prototypes Can

Description: "From Waste to Can"—aerosol can made from 100% post-consumer recycled (PCR) aluminium. The producer applies with its aerosol can made from 100% PCR aluminium. It is the first of its kind containing no primary aluminium at all.

The starting material used is drink can scrap returned by consumers to the collection points for recycling. The collected scrap is pressed, converted into slugs and processed into aerosol cans by Nussbaum using the regular impact extrusion production process. This is what the claim "From Waste to Can" stands for—a can made from scrap/waste only. For this special alloy the patent is pending.

Tool and process innovation are the key to being able to process the high alloy content in the 100% PCR material in the existing process. Our technicians have achieved a 100% replacement of the primary aluminium and an additional reduction in the use of materials. The stronger alloy of the beverage cans makes it possible to manufacture lighter cans with the same performance.

The sustainability goal is perfectly supported thanks to the use of mono material waste, which avoids expensive and complex sorting processes. In addition, the transport routes are short, as the collection point, the aluminium processors and the can manufacturer are located within a 150 km radius.

The use of recycled paper and glass has long been widespread in the private consumer sector. Up until now, recycled metals and aluminum have mainly been reserved for industrial consumers. With its use in the packaging sector, private consumers now also have the opportunity to actively choose packaging made from recycled material when shopping. The existing deposit system for beverage cans enables the aluminum to be reused easily, sorted by type. The additional demand for used beverage cans supports the deposit system and the claim as 100% PCR shows the consumer that the collected material is actually being reused.

The production of recycling aluminium saves 95% of the energy required for the production of virgin material. Using 100% PCR aluminium, 6.84 t of CO_2 are saved per ton of aluminium. Aluminium can be recycled infinitely and around 75% of the ever produced aluminium is still in use today.

中文介绍

9 号罐:

样品罐

产品说明:

"从废物到罐子"——100%由消费后回收(PCR)铝制成的气雾剂罐。生产商使用100%由 PCR 铝制成的气雾剂罐。这是第一款完全不含原(生)铝的气雾罐。

使用的原始材料是消费者扔到回收点的饮料罐废料。努斯鲍姆公司(NUSSBAUM)采用常规的冲击挤压生产工艺将收集到的废罐冲击挤压为块状再加工成气雾罐。这就是"从废料到罐体"的意思——一个只有废料/废物制成的罐子。这种特殊合金的专利正在申请中。

工具和工艺创新是确保现有工艺处理 100% PCR 材料中高合金含量的关键。我们的技术已经实现了100%的原铝替代,并进一步减少了材料的使用。饮料罐的合金强度越高,就越有可能制造出性能相同但重量更轻的罐子。

通过使用单一材料的废弃物,可完美地支持可持续性发展目标,从而避免了昂贵且复杂的分拣过程。此外,由于铝加工商和罐制造商都位于以收集点为中心的 150 公里半径范围内,也缩短了运输路线。

在个人消费领域,回收纸和玻璃早已广泛应用。直到现在,回收金属和铝主要被用于工业领域。随着其在包装行业的应用,个人消费者现在也有机会在购物时主动选择由回收材料制成的包装。现有的饮料罐退瓶系统使铝易于按类型分类回收。对废旧饮料罐的额外需求支持了退瓶系统,而100% PCR 的标志也向消费者表明,收集的材料确实是被重复利用。

与生产原始材料相比,回收铝可节省所需能源的95%。使用100%PCR 铝每吨可节省 68.4 吨二氧化碳。铝可以无限次回收利用,目前已生产的铝大约75%仍在使用中。

2021-9 号罐360 度旋转视频二维码

编号:2021-10

英文介绍

Can No. 10: Save the Earth

Prototypes Can

Description: The producer has partnered with Sun Chemical to produce two self-promotional containers which utilize spot varnish ink technology. The interest/demand for this printing option has become increasing popular with the producer's customers. Contrast in appearance between the matt and gloss promotes the eye-catching shelf presence that marketers embrace. The challenge with this technology stems from the absence of traditional over varnish as the OV is introduced as an additive within the ink. Without over varnish (traditional or OV ink additive), forming the container shape would be extremely difficult. In addition, the OV also protects the container from scratching, chipping or scuffing.

中文介绍

10 号罐:

样品罐

产品说明:

生产商与 SUN CHEMICAL 合作,生产了两款自推广容器,采用了点胶油墨印刷技术。这种印刷方式越来越受到生产商客户的欢迎。哑光和亮光之间的外观对比有助于营销人员对这种引人注目的罐子进行展示。这项技术的挑战源于缺乏传统的覆膜,因为覆膜是作为油墨添加剂引入的。没有传统的覆膜或油墨添加剂,容器成型将是极其困难的。此外,覆膜还可以保护容器免受刮伤、碎裂或磨损。

2021-10 号罐360 度旋转视频二维码

编号：2021-10-1

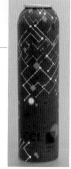

英文介绍

Can No. 10-1: The Matrix

Prototypes Can

Description: The producer has partnered with Sun Chemical to produce two self-promotional containers which utilize spot varnish ink technology. The interest/demand for this printing option has become increasing popular with the producer's customers. Contrast in appearance between the matt and gloss promotes the eye-catching shelf presence that marketers embrace. The challenge with this technology stems from the absence of traditional over varnish as the OV is introduced as an additive within the ink. Without over varnish (traditional or OV ink additive), forming the container shape would be extremely difficult. In addition, the OV also protects the container from scratching, chipping or scuffing.

中文介绍

10-1 号罐：

样品罐

产品说明：

生产商与 SUN CHEMICAL 合作生产了两种自推广容器,采用了点光油技术。这种印刷方法在生产商的客户中越来越受欢迎。哑光和亮光之间的对比可以增强营销人员喜爱的醒目的货架展示效果。这种技术的挑战在于,传统的上光油作为添加剂被加入到油墨中,而没有传统的上光油或上光油添加剂,容器成型是非常困难的。此外,上光油还可以保护容器免受划伤、剥落或擦伤。

2021-10-1 号罐 360 度旋转视频二维码

编号：2021-11

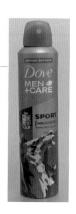

英文介绍

Can No. 11: Dove Men+Care

Marketed Can

Description: The producer and Unilever bring to market a stunning deodorant spray, packaged in aluminum, that celebrates the British & Irish Lions rugby squad.

The producer and Unilever team up to develop a limited edition deodorant spray for the Dove Men+Care brand, available in an infinitely recyclable aerosol can. The limited edition deodorant celebrates the British & Irish Lions, a rugby team comprised of England, Ireland, Scotland and Wales. This spray will be available on shelves in the UK, and celebrates the 2021 Lions tour, which will take place in South Africa during the summer.

The producer and Unilever share a common sense of purpose, with both companies committed to building a healthier planet by helping people live more sustainably. Unilever are on a mission to help reduce waste around the world, so it should come as no surprise that they decide to partner with the producer, to package their product in aluminum: aluminum can be recycled endlessly without any loss of quality, and as a result, 75% of all aluminum ever produced globally is still in use today.

The aluminium aerosol can provides a perfect, 360-degree design canvas which is ideal to celebrate major sports events. The design on the can uses vibrant colors, and strong geographical shapes, resulting in a strong visual impact at point of sales. The boldness of the design is rendered through the producer's high definition printing techniques and capabilities, which bring the graphics to life.

中文介绍

11 号罐：

已上市罐

产品说明：

生产商和联合利华向市场推出了一款绝妙的香体喷雾产品,采用铝制包装,以此庆祝英伦和爱尔兰雄狮橄榄球队。

生产商和联合利华合作为多芬男士护理品牌打造了限量版香体剂,装在可无限回收的气雾剂罐中。这款限量版香体剂是为了庆祝由英格兰、爱尔兰、苏格兰和威尔士组成的英伦和爱尔兰雄狮橄榄球队。这款喷雾剂将在英国出售,以庆祝 2021 年夏季在南非举行的雄狮队巡回赛。

生产商和联合利华有着共同的目标,都致力于建立一个更健康的地球,以帮助人们以更可持续的方式生活。联合利华的使命是帮助减少全球的废弃物,所以他们决定与生产商合作,使用铝包装产品:铝可以被无限回收而不会损失任何质量,因此,全球生产的所有铝材中有75%至今仍在使用。

铝制气雾罐提供了完美的 360 度的设计图案,是庆祝重大体育赛事的理想选择。罐体上的设计使用了鲜艳的色彩和强烈的几何形状,在销售点能够产生强烈的视觉冲击力。这些大胆的设计是通过生产商的高清晰度印刷技术和能力来呈现的,使图案栩栩如生。

2021-11 号罐 360 度旋转视频二维码

编号:2021-12

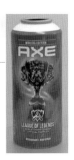

英 文 介 绍

Can No. 12: Axe Market

Marketed Can

Description: The producer and Unilever develop Axe *League of Legends* deodorant for Mexican market.

The producer and Unilever have partnered to develop a deodorant body spray for Axe, the world leading men's grooming brand, in an infinitely recyclable aerosol can. As the first men's grooming sponsor for *League of Legends*, Axe is continuing its effort to align itself with youth-oriented sports, music and culture.

In order to bring to market a can that would resonate with the esport (or electronic sports) competitive video gaming community, it is crucial to develop a stunning design. The obvious choice is to leverage the producer's proprietary Eyeris technique on the aluminum aerosol can. Ideal for printing photographs and highly detailed graphics, Eyeris high-definition printing helps to visualize graphics in extreme details, and to accurately depict colors and texture. With Eyeris, brands are able to engage the consumer through exciting and other/worldly scenes, bringing the consumer into the brand story with graphics that seems so real they captivate the imagination.

Colors do not impact the recyclability of the package: regardless of color or shape, aluminum packaging can be recycled endlessly, and without any loss of quality making it the ideal material for a truly circular economy.

中 文 介 绍

12 号罐:

已上市罐

产品说明:

生产商与联合利华共同为墨西哥市场开发 Axe《英雄联盟》香体剂。

生产商与联合利华合作,为世界领先的男士护理品牌 Axe 开发了一款可无限回收的香体剂喷雾罐。作为《英雄联盟》的首个男士美容赞助商,Axe 将继续努力与面向年轻人的体育、音乐和文化保持一致。

为了向市场推出一款能够与电子竞技电子游戏社区产生共鸣的罐体,令人耳目一新的设计是至关重要的。明智的选择是利用生产商的专利技术 Eyeris 生产铝气雾剂罐。Eyeris 的高清打印非常适合打印照片和清晰的图形,它能在微小细节中可视化图形,并准确描绘颜色和纹理。借助 Eyeris,品牌能够通过令人兴奋和超凡脱俗的场景吸引消费者,用看似真实的图形吸引他们的想象力,将他们带入品牌故事。

颜色不会影响包装的可回收性,无论颜色或形状如何,铝包装都可以无限次地被回收利用,并且没有任何质量损失,使其成为循环经济中的理想材料。

2021-12 号罐 360 度旋转视频二维码

编号:2021-13

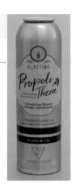

英文介绍

Can No. 13: Elastine Propoli Thera Volumizing Mousse

Marketed Can

Description: P613C Fareva Richmond Can—0383 Elastine Propoli Thera Volumizing Mousse 142 g, 45 mm×150 mm, featuring our round shoulder, clear base coating applied over a brushed aluminum base can, dry offset printed graphics, gloss over varnish, and 2Q pressure rating.

For this example, the customer is developing a new product line for beauty and cosmetics use. The customer provides a very good prototype can which is done via shrink sleeve and digital printing. We are asked to create our printed can to match their prototype. Our ink vendor INX does a great job at interpreting what is needed by the customer. Another complexity in color development is the use of transparent and opaque inks for this project. Our customer wants to allow some of the brushed can marks to show through some colors, but not in others.

The graphics are very complex and very fine detail in the "Propolis" round logo at the top of the front panel, and the bee graphic. We use our dot gain curves to make sure the screened watermark pattern held open and reproduced correctly. The center opaque beige logo on the front of the can and the white background in the circular logo make this a very attractive can.

Our production team do an excellent job at making sure this aerosol aluminum can meet the customer's expectations. We also hold a "virtual" press approval with the client, just to make sure they are happy with our print quality—"COVID-19" had given us a very challenging past 18 months. Also, thanks to our digital platemaking, we are able to make very accurate plates and hold those screened graphics as the customer wanted.

中文介绍

13 号罐:

已上市罐

产品说明:

P613C Fareva Richmond 罐具有 0383 Elastine Propoli Thera 摩丝 142 克、45 mm×150 mm、圆肩、涂在拉丝铝罐上的透明底涂层、干胶印图形、光油以及 2Q 压力等级。

对于这个样品,客户正在开发一条用于美容和化妆品的新产品线。客户提供了一个非常好的原型罐,这是通过收缩套膜和数字印刷完成的。我们被要求制作与他们的原型相匹配的印刷罐。我们的油墨供应商 INX 在理解客户需求方面做得很好。色彩发展的另一个复杂性是透明和不透明油墨的使用。我们的客户希望罐体的拉丝效果能在某些颜色中显现出来,而在其他颜色中则不显示。

在罐子主视面顶部的"蜂胶"圆形标志和蜜蜂图案中,图形非常复杂,细节非常精细。我们使用网点增益曲线确保网点水印图案处于打开状态并正确呈现。罐体正面中心的不透明米色标志和圆形标志的白色背景,让人觉得这是一个非常吸引人的罐体。

我们的生产团队在确保这种铝气雾剂罐可以满足客户的期望方面做得非常出色。我们还与客户进行了"虚拟"印刷审批,确保他们对我们的印刷质量感到满意——"COVID-19"在过去的 18 个月给我们带来了非常大的挑战。此外,得益于我们的数字制版技术,我们能够制作非常精确的版型,并根据客户的需要保留那些网点水印图案。

2021-13 号罐 360 度旋转视频二维码

编号:2021-14

英文介绍

Can No. 14: Peace Eyes on Me

Prototypes Can

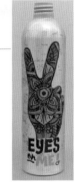

Description: P736C Peace Eyes on Me cosmetic bottle—16 fl oz 59 mm×216 mm, featuring our round shoulder and our new 28-410 threaded neck, clear base coating applied over a brushed aluminum base can, dry offset printed graphics, gloss over varnish. This prototype can represents our entry into the cosmetic pump aluminum bottle market. We are seeing demand for sustainable packaging opportunities, this being one of those markets. Our engineering, sales, marketing, and graphics staff work together to bring this concept from the drawing table to finished product.

The graphics are done by our in-house graphics team using bright colors which our ink vendor INX do a great job at interpreting what was needed by our staff. Another complexity in color development is the use of transparent and opaque inks for this project. The white and black contrast with the other very bright transparent colors create a very unique style which should help our potential customer base fully understand our 9-color printing capability and razor sharp graphic reproduction using our digital plates.

Our production team do an excellent job at making sure this aluminum pump bottle met expectations. Also, thanks to our digital platemaking, we are able to make very accurate plates and hold those screened graphics as the customer wanted.

中文介绍

14 号罐:

样品罐

产品说明:

  P736C 和平之眼化妆品罐,具有 16 盎司、59 mm×216 mm、圆肩和新的 28~410 螺纹肩、透明的底涂层应用在拉丝铝罐、干胶印图形以及光油。这款创新型罐子可以代表我们开始进入化妆品铝泵罐市场。我们看到了对可持续包装产品的需求,这是其中一个市场。我们的工程、市场、营销和设计人员共同努力,将这个概念从图纸推进到成品。

  图案是由我们的内部图形设计团队使用鲜艳的颜色完成的,我们的油墨供应商 INX 在了解我们员工的需求方面做了大量工作。色彩处理的另一个复杂性是透明和不透明油墨的使用。黑白对比与其他明亮的透明颜色创造了一个非常独特的风格,这应该有助于潜在客户充分了解我们的 9 色印刷能力和使用数字技术形成的快速制版能力。

  我们的生产团队在确保铝泵罐达到预期方面做得非常出色。此外,由于我们使用数字制版,我们能够制作非常精确的版型,并根据客户的需要保留那些网点水印图案。

2021-14 号罐 360 度旋转视频二维码

五、2020 年国际铝气雾罐竞赛参赛罐

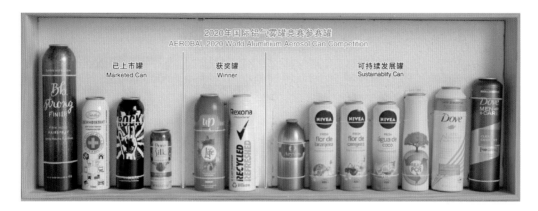

罐编号从左至右分别是:3,9,8,5,11,10,12,4-1,4-2,4-3,2,6,1

编号:2020-1

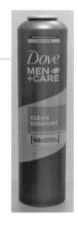

英文介绍

Can No. 1: Dove Men & Care

Sustainability Can

Description: A light-weight aerosol can with 20% weight reduction manufactured with a new patented alloy (Neucan 3.1). This patented alloy allows the use of 25% PCR material or even more, depending on the composition/quality of the PCR material (Designed to Recycle). The significant weight loss is achieved by reducing the wall thickness and slightly modifying the shape of the shoulder compared to the previous shape.

Challenge: The reduced wall thickness makes the can more susceptible to dents during packing and transporting.

Solution: Introducing new packaging process-layer wide packaging. Cans are placed on pallets instead of packed in bundles. Packing is fully automatic. Savings of this new packing process are: 15% more cans fit on a pallet, 15% more pallets fit on a truck, 15% less warehouse space needed. Three times 15% is another important aspect of sustainability besides less aluminium and PCR content.

中文介绍

1 号罐:

可持续发展罐

产品说明:

一种轻量化气雾剂罐,采用新型专利合金(Neucan 3.1)制造,重量减轻了 20%。这种专利合金允许使用 25% 甚至更多的回收再利用材料,这取决于回收再利用材料的成分/质量(专为循环而设计)。与以前的形状相比,通过减少壁厚和稍微改变肩部的形状,罐的重量明显减轻。

挑战:壁厚的减少使罐子在包装和运输过程中更容易产生凹痕。

解决方案:引入新的包装工艺——分层包装。罐子被放在托盘上,而不是捆扎包装。包装是全自动的。这种新的包装过程节省之处包括:托盘上可以多装 15% 的罐子、卡车上可以多装 15% 的托盘、可以节省 15% 的仓库空间。

除了减少铝用量和利用回收材料外,以上 3 个方面的 15% 是可持续性发展的另一个重要方面。

2020-1 号罐 360 度旋转视频二维码

编号:2020-2

英文介绍

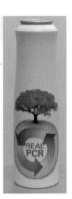

Can No. 2: Patented Alloy and Real PCR

Sustainability Can

Description: Alloy is good.

Alloy and real PCR is better.

Up to 60 per cent real PCR is brilliant!

The target of this new and patented alloy was: reduce weight by 20 per cent and more, use real PCR with up to 60 per cent, cradle to cradle, allow complex shapes with zero tolerance in specification and quality.

The idea of this concept is that customers can decide the percentage of PCR material used—depending on their strategy and requirements. The solution is only possible by joining forces with external experts and metallurgists to design this new slug solution—giving the customers the mentioned advantages.

Solutions shown are:

can with 25 per cent real PCR

can with 60 per cent real PCR

中文介绍

2 号罐:

可持续发展罐

产品说明：

合金是一种非常好的材料。

合金和回收再利用材料结合更好。

高达60%的真正回收再利用材料更是极好的！

这种新型专利合金的目标是：重量减少20%以上，并使用高达60%的闭环再生材料，允许制造具有零公差规格和质量的复杂形状。

这个概念的理念是客户可以根据自己的策略和需求决定使用回收再利用材料的比例。只有通过与外部专家和冶金学家联合设计这种新型的铝片解决方案，才能为客户提供上述优势。

展示的解决方案包括：含有25%回收再利用材料的罐子与含有60%回收再利用材料的罐子。

2020-2号罐360度旋转视频二维码

编号：2020-3

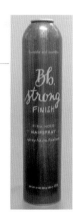

英 文 介 绍

Can No. 3: Estée Lauder Bumble & Bumble Strong Finish Hairspray Marketed Can

Description: This innovative product is a blend of resin and transform that delivers a strong, long lasting hold with a modern finish. To complement this awesome product, the container is designed to stand out on store and studio shelves. Achieving customers' expectations is challenging, the producer incorporated split-well ink technologies to deliver smooth colour transitions without the pixelated look of a half tone screen. In addition to the smooth transitions, colour saturation is enhanced with an overall screen to help achieve that "darker edge" the customer is looking for.

Due to the abundance of colour within this can design, selective edging is done around the text in efforts to maintain legibility of the front and back panel copy, which aids in promoting the brand. The Bumble & Bumble Strong Finish Hairspray is a great success: product, packaging, functionality that have received many positive reviews.

中 文 介 绍

3号罐：

已上市罐

产品说明：

这款创新产品是树脂和改造混合而成,具有现代风格的饰面,经久耐用。为了完成这个极佳的产品,该罐的设计旨在让其在商店的货架和设计室的展示架上脱颖而出。实现客户的期望是具有挑战性的,生产商采用了分段式墨水技术,以提供色彩的平滑过渡,而不会出现半色调显示的像素化外观。除了色彩的平滑过渡外,显示的色彩饱和度整个也得到了增强,以帮助客户寻找到"更暗的临界点"。

由于这个罐体设计中有丰富的颜色,为了保持前后罐体表面的清晰度,在文本周围做了选择性的边缘,这有助于提升品牌形象。Bumble & Bumble 强力定型发胶获得很大成功:其产品、包装、功能得到了许多好评。

2020-3 号罐 360 度旋转视频二维码

编号:2020-4-1

英文介绍

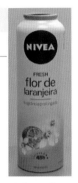

Can No. 4-1: Nivea Senses

Sustainability Can

Description: The Nivea senses project available on the market under the new slim aero Nivea design, in the versions fresh orange, cherry blossom and coconut water are strategically designed to deliver a sustainability gain with a significant weight reduction within the aluminium cans. The new shape designed for this project and the weight reduction of the cans are supported by an advanced aluminium alloy, giving all the characteristics that a great aerosol can needs. Besides the alloy and design, the printing process is also meticulously thought to deliver an outstanding result of 11 colours for the fresh orange and cherry blossom versions and 9 colours for the coconut water version. The sustainability compromise into the entire slim aero project will generate an annual reduction of more than 300 tons of aluminium. Together with the characteristic new shape of the can and sophisticated printing gives to the final senses version product and the brand a distinctive and impressive overall appearance at the point of sale. To deliver this project Beiersdorf Latam Team has the producer as its strategic partner.

中文介绍

4-1 号罐:

可持续发展罐

产品说明:

市场上的 Nivea 感官项目采用了新的纤细流线型 Nivea 设计,有鲜橙、樱花和椰子三个版本,其战略设计是通过显著减轻铝罐的重量来实现可持续发展。为这个项目设计的新形状和轻量化的罐体由一种先进的铝合金组成,其提供了优异的气雾剂罐所需的所有特性。除了合金材料和设计,印刷过程也经过精心考虑,为新鲜橙子和樱花版本提供了 11 种颜色,为椰子版本提供了 9 种颜色。整个纤细流线型产品设计项目对可持续性发展的承诺是每年将减少 300 多吨铝。加上独特的新形状和复杂的印刷工艺,最终的产品和品牌在销售点具有独特而令人印象深刻的整体外观。为了完成这个项目,拜尔斯道夫拉丁团队将制作人作为其战略合作伙伴。

2020-4-1 号罐 360 度旋转视频二维码

编号:2020-4-2

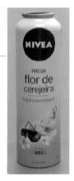

英 文 介 绍

Can No. 4-2: Nivea Senses

Sustainability Can

Description: The Nivea senses project available on the market under the new slim aero Nivea design, in the versions fresh orange, cherry blossom and coconut water are strategically designed to deliver a sustainability gain with a significant weight reduction within the aluminium cans. The new shape designed for this project and the weight reduction of the cans are supported by an advanced aluminium alloy, giving all the characteristics that a great aerosol can needs. Besides the alloy and design, the printing process is also meticulously thought to deliver an outstanding result of 11 colours for the fresh orange and cherry blossom versions and 9 colours for the coconut water version. The sustainability compromise into the entire slim aero project will generate an annual reduction of more than 300 tons of aluminium. Together with the characteristic new shape of the can and sophisticated printing gives to the final senses version product and the brand a distinctive and impressive overall appearance at the point of sale. To deliver this project Beiersdorf Latam Team has the producer as its strategic partner.

中 文 介 绍

4-2 号罐:

可持续发展罐

产品说明:

　　市场上的 Nivea 感官项目采用了新的纤细流线型 Nivea 设计,有鲜橙、樱花和椰子三个版本,其战略设计是通过显著减轻铝罐的重量来实现可持续发展。为这个项目设计的新形状和轻量化的罐体由一种先进的铝合金组成,其提供了优异的气雾剂罐所需的所有特性。除了合金材料和设计,印刷过程也经过精心考虑,为新鲜橙子和樱花版本提供了 11 种颜色,为椰子版本提供了9种颜色。整个纤细流线型产品设计项目对可持续性发展的承诺是每年将减少300多吨铝。加上独特的新形状和复杂的印刷工艺,最终的产品和品牌在销售点具有独特而令人印象深刻的整体外观。为了完成这个项目,拜尔斯道夫拉丁团队将制作人作为其战略合作伙伴。

2020-4-2 号罐 360 度旋转视频二维码

编号:2020-4-3

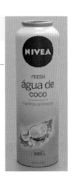

英文介绍

Can No. 4-3: Nivea Senses

Sustainability Can

Description: The Nivea Senses project available on the market under the new slim aero Nivea design, in the versions fresh orange, cherry blossom and coconut water are strategically designed to deliver a sustainability gain with a significant weight reduction within the aluminium cans. The new shape designed for this project and the weight reduction of the cans are supported by an advanced aluminium alloy, giving all the characteristics that a great aerosol can needs. Besides the alloy and design, the printing process is also meticulously thought to deliver an outstanding result of 11 colours for the fresh orange and cherry blossom versions and 9 colours for the coconut water version. The sustainability compromise into the entire Slim Aero Project will generate an annual reduction of more than 300 tons of aluminium. Together with the characteristic new shape of the can and sophisticated printing gives to the final senses version product and the brand a distinctive and impressive overall appearance at the point of sale. To deliver this project Beiersdorf Latam Team has the producer as its strategic partner.

中文介绍

4-3 号罐:

可持续发展罐

产品说明:

市场上的 Nivea 感官项目采用了新的纤细流线型 Nivea 设计,有鲜橙、樱花和椰子三个版本,其战略设计是通过显著减轻铝罐的重量来实现可持续发展。为这个项目设计的新形状和轻量化的罐体由一种先进的铝合金组成,其提供了优异的气雾剂罐所需的所有特性。除了合金材料和设计,印刷过程也经过精心考虑,为新鲜橙子和樱花版本提供了 11 种颜色,为椰子版本提供了9种颜色。整个纤细流线型产品设计项目对可持续性发展的承诺是每年将减少300多吨铝。加上独特的新形状和复杂的印刷,最终的产品和品牌在销售点具有独特而令人印象深刻的整体外观。为了完成这个项目,拜尔斯道夫拉丁团队将制作人作为其战略合作伙伴。

2020-4-3 号罐 360 度旋转视频二维码

编号:2020-5

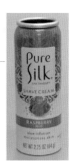

英文介绍

Can No. 5: Puresilk Raspberry

Marketed Can

Description: The Puresilk Raspberry shave utilises a variety challenging of printing techniques including an intricate background design.

The use of opaque and transparent inks systems accentuate the brushed aluminium substrate.

中文介绍

5 号罐:

已上市罐

产品说明:

Puresilk 覆盆子剃须产品采用多种具有挑战性的印刷技术,包括复杂的背景设计。

不透明和透明油墨系统的使用突出了拉丝铝基材。

2020-5 号罐 360 度旋转视频二维码

编号:2020-6

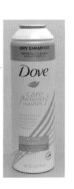

英文介绍

Can No. 6: Dove 5.0 oz Dry Shampoo

Sustainability Can

Description: This can uses an advanced alloy that weighs 14% less than the standard 1070 alloy and also uses up to 25% recycled content.

With a large distribution this sustainable impact is notable.

中文介绍

6号罐：

可持续发展罐

产品说明：

这种罐使用一种先进的合金，重量比标准的1070合金轻14％，并且使用高达25％的可回收材料。

由于分布广泛，这种可持续影响是显著的。

2020-6号罐360度旋转视频二维码

编号：2020-8

英文介绍

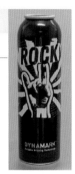

Can No. 8: Dynamark

Marketed Can

Description: Your package is the most important billboard, and thanks to the producer's new breakthrough printing capabilities, you can create more exciting promotions than ever before. Dynamark TM variable printing technology allows brands to add graphic variety to their cans without introducing the expensive and tie-consuming operational challenges of the past.

You have the ability to add up to 12 different graphics to your print run at a reasonable cost. Dynamark TM can be used to launch social engagement campaigns, print limited time promotions and increase brand loyalty and sales. This new innovation has been years in the making and the producer is excited to finally make it available to the market.

中文介绍

8号罐：

已上市罐

产品说明：

包装是一个产品最重要的广告牌，由于生产者在印刷能力上的新突破，你可以开展比以往任何时候都更令人兴奋的提升行动。Dynamark TM可变印刷技术允许品牌在不引入过去昂贵和耗时的操作挑战的情况下，为他们的罐体添加可变化的图案。

您可以用合理的成本添加多达12种不同的图案。Dynamark TM可用于发起社会参与活动、印刷限时促销、提高品牌忠诚度和销售量。这项新的创新已经酝酿了数年，终于由生产商将其推向了市场。

2020-8 号罐 360 度旋转视频二维码

编号:2020-9

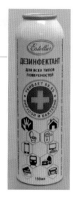

英 文 介 绍

Can No. 9: Estellar

Marketed Can

Description: The producer has been producing aluminium aerosol cans for one of its Russian customers for a long time. "Estellar" branded disinfectant spray of Aerostar Contract Aerosol Filling Company has been brought to the market in a short time thanks to both parties' extraordinary efforts during these COVID-19 high-times. The producer feels that taking a different approach or responsibility during these difficult times is also very important. Shaping new cans, can help to gain better market shares. Trying to reduce the weight of the can is also an important step toward success for sustainability. There is no doubt that reducing the weight of can help to lower the carbon footprint which potentially allows a cleaner planet in the future. Designing with simplicity, clear printing, and specified colour aimed to accommodate only the needs of the end-user by focusing on timely decision making i. e. having a disinfectant spray ready. The artwork has been expressing itself effortlessly and provides necessary instructions to the consumers with its smoothly printed high-quality infographics while disregarding excessive designs or innovations. The producer is very proud of his employees during the pandemic who promptly made this product available to fulfil a significant healthcare need. The producer once again has proven its innovative and flexible approach to fulfil the market demands with a non-traditional way.

中 文 介 绍

9 号罐:

已上市罐

产品说明:

该生产商长期以来一直为其中的一家俄罗斯客户生产铝制气雾剂罐。在新冠疫情高发时期,双方付出了非凡的努力,在短时间内将 Aerostar Contract Aerosol 灌装公司的"Estellar"牌消毒喷雾推向市场。生产商觉得在困难时期采取不同的方法或承担不同的责任是非常重要的。制造新的罐体有助于获得更好的市场份额。尝试减轻罐子的重量也是企业迈向可持续发展的重要一步。毫无疑问,罐子重量的减轻有助于降低碳足迹,这可能会使未来的地球更清洁。简洁的设计、清晰的印刷和特定的颜色,重点是及时决策,旨在满足最终用户的需求,例如准备好消毒喷雾。艺术品可以轻松地展示自己,并以其流畅的高质量图案为消费者提供必要的指导,无需过多的设计或创新。生产商对其员工在疫情防控期间迅速提供该产品以满足重大医疗保健需求感到非常自豪。生产商再次证明了其创新性和灵活性,以非传统的方式满足市场需求。

2020-9 号罐 360 度旋转视频二维码

编号:2020-10

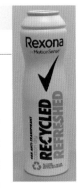

英文介绍

Can No. 10: Rexona Recycled Refreshed Sustainability Can

Description: Manufactured with a new patented alloy, with 25 per cent real PCR inclusion (joint effort of manufacturer and brand). The can is 14 per cent lighter than the previous design due to use of alloy, layerwide packaging and slight modification of shape. Furthermore powder coating is used as internal lacquer and on top of that is the can only partially lacquered (50 per cent). The ecological advantage of powder coating: no VOC is emitted when applied inside the can and the overspray is reused, sustainability at its best!

中文介绍

10 号罐:

可持续发展罐

产品说明:

这种罐采用一种新的专利合金制造,含有 25% 的可回收再利用材料(由制造商和品牌方的共同努力的结果)。由于使用合金、分层包装和使形状轻微改变,该罐体比之前的设计轻 14%。此外,粉末涂料被用作内涂层,最重要的是罐子只需要部分涂料(50%)。粉末涂料具有明显的生态优势:在罐内使用时不会排放挥发性有机化合物,多余的喷雾可重复使用,是最具可持续发展的!

2020-10 号罐 360 度旋转视频二维码

编号:2020-11

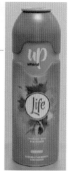

英 文 介 绍

Can No.11: Half Moon

Marketed Can

Description:

The producer's Tunisian customer who is strong in perfume business in Tunis, decides to develop their own deodorant spray brand after they had presented several famous French deodorant spray brands in Tunis as distributor. That's why they want to create a special deodorant spray line with 4 different fragrances. They pay almost the same attention at the packaging as the fragrance because that would be their first own branded body spray project. As there are almost the same types of aluminium cans in the market, they look for something attractive and innovative. That is their main reason why they contact the producer for a special type of aluminium can options for 200 mL. After several simulation trials with different type of cans, the producer offers an innovative aluminium can which has 360° embossed shaping with oriented printing technology. Compared to the aluminium aerosol cans with traditional standard shapes, 360° embossed shaping with oriented printing technology gives a unique shaped deformation around the circumference of the aluminium can and this enables a special 360° deformed & printed area apart from the flat surface of the can where you can highlight your brand or logo.

The result is very fascinating and the customer has no worries about counterfeiting since this technology and the special mould called "Half Moon Emboss Shape" has been developed by the producer. This unique embossing technology provides below vital points to the customers:

Brighten up your brand with the unique technology!

Protect your brand against counterfeiting!

Differentiate your brand from the competitors with innovation!

Wide range of shapes!

Custom design shape development!

Available diameters for 450 mm, 500 mm, 530 mm!

Available options for 150 mL, 200 mL, 250 mL!

中 文 介 绍

11 号罐:

已上市罐

产品说明:

生产商的突尼斯客户在突尼斯有很强大的香水业务,他们作为经销商参观了几个著名的法国香体剂喷雾品牌后,决定开发自己的香体剂品牌。这就是为什么他们想要创造一个系列的特殊香体剂喷雾产品,包括 4 种不同的香味。

他们对香体剂的包装和产品一样关注,因为这是他们第一个自己品牌的香体喷雾项目。

由于市场上的铝罐几乎都是相同的,他们努力寻找一些有吸引力和创新的东西。这是他们联系生产商的主要原因,他们需要一种特殊类型的 200 mL 铝罐。在对不同类型的罐体进行模拟试验后,生产商提供了一种创新的铝罐,该罐具有 360°浮雕成型和定向印刷技术。与传统标准形状的铝气雾罐相比,360°浮雕成型与定向印刷技术使铝罐形成独特的形状,这使得除了可以突出品牌或标志的平面图案外,还可以实现特殊的 360°变形,并且留出印刷区域。

生产商开发了被称为"半月浮雕"的技术和特殊的模具,这是非常有吸引力的,客户不用担心产品被假冒。这种独特的浮雕技术为客户提供以下关键优势:

用独特的技术点亮您的品牌!

保护您的品牌免受假冒!

用创新让你的品牌从竞争对手中脱颖而出!

可供选择的各种形状!

造型可定制设计!

可提供不同直径选项 45 mm、50 mm、53 mm!

可提供多种容量选项 150 mL、200 mL、250 mL!

2020-11 号罐 360 度旋转视频二维码

编号:2020-12

英文介绍

Can No. 12: No Gas

Sustainability Can

Description:

Thanks to the producer's experience in the production of 360° embossed aluminium cans and 3 awards for this technology since 2015, they wanted to produce also a standard aluminium can last year in 45 mm diam which had 20 mm opening and was used for no gas products. Due to the special opening apart from the standard 1″ aerosol cans, the required valve and also the valve crimping process is easier for the customers compared to the standard aerosol filling.

The high demand placed on this product in a short time leed them to have the idea to improve the same product with an innovative touch. After several trials on 45 mm×105 mm and 20 mm opening aluminium can, they applied their 360° embossing technology to this very small aluminium can which worked fine. There are different types of embossed cans in the market as well as several aluminium can producers for the standard aluminium cans with 20 mm opening, however, there is not any such small aluminium can with embossing technology in the market.

The producer aims to produce this unique small embossed aluminium cans for the premium branded perfumes as well as semi pharma cosmetic products such as mouth freshener sprays, sanitizer sprays, freshening spray colognes etc. , which are filled into aluminium can and does not require gas filling inside.

中文介绍

12 号罐：

可持续发展罐

产品说明：

　　由于生产商在生产 360°浮雕铝罐方面的经验以及自 2015 年以来该技术获得的 3 个奖项，他们去年还想生产 45 mm 直径的标准铝罐，其开口为 20 mm，用于无气体产品。与标准的 1 英寸口径气雾剂罐不同，该罐有特殊的开口，与标准气雾剂灌装相比，该罐所需的阀门和阀门压接过程对客户来说更容易。

　　在短时间内对该产品的高需求使他们产生了以创新的方式改进同一产品的想法。在 45 mm×105 mm 且口径 20 mm 的铝罐上进行几次试验后，他们将 360°浮雕技术应用到这个非常小的铝罐上，效果良好。市场上有不同类型的浮雕罐，也有几家铝罐生产商生产 20 mm 口径的标准铝罐，然而，市场上还没有这种带有浮雕技术的小铝罐。

　　生产商的目标是生产这种独特的小型浮雕铝罐，用于高档品牌香水和半医药化妆品如口腔清新剂喷雾、消毒剂喷雾、清新喷雾古龙水等，这些产品可以直接灌装在铝罐中，不需要填充气体。

2020-12 号罐 360 度旋转视频二维码

六、2019年国际铝气雾罐竞赛参赛罐

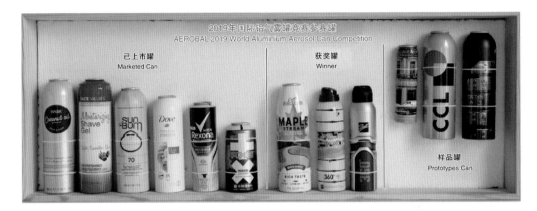

罐编号从左至右分别是:9,8,7,2,5,6,10,11,11-1,1,3,4

编号:2019-1

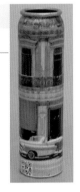

英文介绍

Can No. 1: Silkscreen Print on Aluminium Cans

Prototypes Can

Description: The difference between silkscreen print and dry offset print is the outstanding opacity of the colours and the haptic sensation. To carve out the contrasts of the car's colour, multiple layers between of colours have been applied. On top of the bright red of the car—black has been printed to give the car's lacquer a three dimensional look. And as the faces on the balustrade show it is also possible to create extremely fine details in silkscreen print as well, comparable to offset print.

This prototype shows that various printing techniques can be adapted to an aluminum aerosol can.

中文介绍

1号罐:

样品罐

产品说明:

丝网印刷和干胶印的区别在于颜色的不透明性和触觉感知。为了突出汽车颜色的对比,使用了多层颜色。在汽车的亮红色车顶上用黑色印刷赋予汽车一个三维的外观。正如栏杆上的脸所显示的那样,丝网印刷也可以创造出非常精细的细节,与胶印相当。

这个样品罐表明,各种印刷技术都可以运用于铝制气雾罐。

2019-1 号罐 360 度旋转视频二维码

编号：**2019-2**

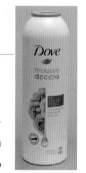

英文介绍

Can No. 2: Dove Shower Mousse Rose Oil

Marketed Can

Description: The can manufacturer uses state of the art artwork separation and special screens to realize such perfect roses. The blossom has an outstanding definition of the image. To ensure such definition a new high-resolution quality computer to plate device is used to create the printing plate. The print specialists build-up the screens in such a unique way that the result is a photorealistic print in HD quality. The secret behind these photorealistic roses is the modular build-up of the screen dots and their specific geometry combined with multiple printing. An image is so real that you're about to smell the scent of the roses. Also, a high-density ink is used to render the very fine, soft yet short transition at the drop of the oil. The can's overall clean appearance achieves a successful promise of the content.

中文介绍

2 号罐：

已上市罐

产品说明：

　　罐体制造商使用了最先进的工艺分离技术和特殊的网版制作出如此完美的玫瑰图案。花朵的图像清晰度非常好。为了确保这样的清晰度,一台新的高分辨率计算机制版设备被用来制作印版。印刷专家以一种独特的方式构建网版,结果呈现了高清质量的印刷效果。这些逼真的玫瑰背后的秘密是网点的模块化构建和通过多次印刷形成的特定的几何形状。画面如此逼真,以至于都要闻到玫瑰的香味了。此外,高密度油墨用于在油滴处呈现非常精细、柔软而短暂的过渡效果。

　　该罐的整体清新的外观实现了对内容的成功阐释。

2019-2 号罐 360 度旋转视频二维码

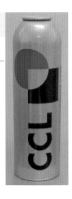

编号：2019-3

英文介绍

Can No. 3: Mirror Appearance Ink

Prototypes Can

Description: CCL Container in partnership with sun Chemical produces a self-promotional can incorporating a mirror-like silver ink. In the past, this brilliant appearance was limited to base-coating which is a flood coating of the can. This limited the design and in certain cases does not deliver the brand intention.

Demand for a foil-like appearance has been driven by CPG's currently executing their designs in the flexographic market as a shrink sleeve or label. Now, the ability to now directly print this appearance on an aluminium container will reduce overall cost and provide new design for concepts.

中文介绍

3 号罐：

样品罐

产品说明：

CCL 灌装公司与太阳化学公司合作生产了一种用于自我宣传的罐体,其表面具有像镜子一样的银涂层。在过去,这种出色的外观仅限于底涂层,这是一种对罐子的满涂。这限制了设计,在某些情况下也无法传达品牌意图。

对箔状外观的需求是由 CPG 推动的。他们通常在柔版印刷市场以收缩套筒或标签的形式执行其设计。如今,直接在铝容器上打印这种外观图案的能力将降低总体成本,并提供新的设计概念。

2019-3 号罐 360 度旋转视频二维码

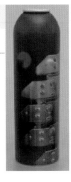

编号：2019-4

英文介绍

Can No. 4: Spot Varnish—Gloss/Matte

Prototypes Can

Description: CCL Container in partnership with Sun Chemical produces a self-promotional can incorporating a gloss and matte appearance. Achieving this appearance has been technically challenging for mono-bloc because the over-varnish in the past has provided a slip mechanism for the shoulder/finishing of the can and to resist marking during transit.

Overcoming this challenge requires building a slip function into the ink as well as producing an ink that can handle being shaped and shipped without scratching, chipping, or scuffing. Demand for gloss and matte on the same container has been driven by the desire to reduce manufacturing costs by the CPG's currently covering aluminium containers with shrink sleeves incorporating special appearances such as gloss and matte. This development may also drive CPG's with product lines that don't have the budget to use special effects to now entertain this option in order to gain more noticeability on the shelf.

中 文 介 绍

4 号罐：

样品罐

产品说明：

CCL 灌装公司与太阳化学公司合作生产了一种用于自我宣传的罐体,结合了亮光和哑光外观。实现这种外观对于单个罐体来说在技术上具有挑战性,因为过去光泽的表面涂料为罐体的肩部/表面提供了润滑机制,并在运输过程中减少刮伤。

要克服这一挑战,就需要在涂料中加入润滑功能,并生产出一种涂料,确保罐体在成型和运输时不会被刮伤、碎裂或磨损。为了降低制造成本,CPG 目前在铝制容器上覆盖了包括亮光和哑光等特殊外观的收缩套,从而推动了对同一容器特殊表面如亮光和哑光的需求。这一发展也可能促使那些没有预算的产品线的 CPG 认真考虑这个选择,以便其产品在货架上获得更多关注。

2019-4 号罐 360 度旋转视频二维码

编号：**2019-5**

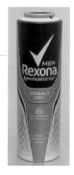

英 文 介 绍

Can No. 5: Rexona Men Motion Sense

Marketed Can

Description: Packaging is very important aspect of a product not only by the way it looks but also its functionality. Sustainability recently has become yet another dimension that requires the attention of packaging industry. Understanding life cycle impact of the product is the key to assess product sustainability.

Having had the life cycle impact of aerosol cans, aluminium is the major issue to tackle for product environmental sustainability. To that end, we adapt design for sustainability philosophy where we manage to develop a new aluminium alloy to produce new at reduced weight for the same volume. Such reduction in weight brings about sizeable reduction in many environmental impacts assessed by using Life Cycle Assessment (LCA) methodology. In this context, aerosol cans are produced with "Magnesium-Manganese-Aluminium alloy" raw material as an alternative to the 99.7% and 99.5% pure aluminium raw material been has used for many years in the sector. These new innovative raw materials meet the mechanical properties required by the standards with thinner wall thickness and offer important opportunities for sustainability.

In this project, which is developed with Unilever and raw material suppliers, Omega shaped cans (45 mm diameter, 145 mm height) are produced with MgMnAluminium alloy slugs and we save about 3.57 grams of raw material for per unit. According to Life Cycle Assessment (LCA) by Metsims, reduction of around 8% is observed in the carbon footprint especially thanks to these savings. Not only reduction in carbon footprint effect, but also many environmental impacts such as global warming potential, ozone layer depletion and fresh water eco-toxicity have improved from 6.5% to 12.3%. Considering the investment costs needed to eliminate the impact of the carbon footprint and environmental effects, it is provided cost reduction 0.024 euro per can for Omega shaped cans.

中文介绍

5 号罐:

已上市罐

产品说明:

包装是一个产品非常重要的方面,不仅体现在外观上,而且体现在功能上。可持续性最近已经成为包装行业关注的一个维度。了解产品的生命周期是评估产品可持续性的关键。

通过对影响气雾罐的生命周期因素进行分析,铝是解决产品对环境可持续性的主要因素。为此,我们根据可持续发展的理念调整了设计,开发了一种新的铝合金,以减轻罐体相同容量时的重量。使用生命周期评估方法,罐子重量的减轻大大减少了对环境对影响。在这种情况下,用"镁锰合金铝"原料生产的气雾剂罐,替代了该行业多年来使用的 99.7% 和 99.5% 纯铝原料。这些创新的原材料使用使罐壁更薄,能够满足标准化生产要求的机械性能,为可持续发展提供了重要的机会。

在联合利华和原材料供应商共同开发的项目中,Omega 形罐(直径 45 mm,高 145 mm)采用镁锰铝合金生产,每罐可节省原材料约 3.57 克。根据 Metsims 的生命周期评估法,由于节省了原材料,碳足迹减少了约 8%。不仅减少碳足迹效应,全球变暖趋势、臭氧层损耗、淡水生态毒性等环境影响,这些诸多环境影响也从 6.5% 改善到 12.3%。由于考虑到消除碳足迹影响和环境影响所需的投资成本,规定每个 Omega 形罐的成本要降低 0.024 欧元。

2019-5 号罐 360 度旋转视频二维码

编号:2019-6

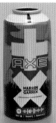

英文介绍

Can No. 6: Unilever Axe Martin Garrix Black Light Can

Marketed Can

Description:

One of the many strengths the producer brings to the table as a supplier is the knowledge shared across divisions and various metal can making. The producer's beverage division previously develops a black light lithography solution for a large beer customer and bases on the learning from this project, the producer's aerosol packaging division explored this printing technique. They are able to create a slightly evolved variation of black light printing, and believe it would be a great innovation for an aerosol can, should the right customer and project present itself.

Enter the Martin Garrix limited edition Unilever Axe can. Axe's brillian partnership with Martin Garrix, the Dutch DJ and producer, provides the perfect opportunity to bring black light to life on an aerosol can. The 22-year-old artist recently released a single, *Ocean with Khalid*, and he's headlined several of the world's biggest music festivals and even performed at the Winter Olympics Closing Ceremony in South Korea. In short, Martin Garrix speaks to the perfect demographic for Axe. In a press release from Unilever, Rik Strubel, Axe's global vice president says, "Music seems a natural extension of the Axe brand. We're all about attraction and music has the power to bring people together, so we know we want to do more in that space. Garrix is a great example to young guys—he's achieved so much at such a young age and boasts natural confidence that is so on brand with Axe. We're super honoured that he's joining Axe Music as our ambassador and we're looking forward to the amazing things we'll do together."

When the producer's team in San Luis Potosi learns of this partnership, they are eager and enthused, as one of Garrix's most successful markets is Mexico. The promotion and coverage of his live shows depict an environment where Garrix literally illuminates the night with his branded lighting. It becomes clear that there is no better way to extend this branding to his shelf presence than to mimic that illumination on an aerosol can. The producer and Unilever set to work to incorporate the producer's black light technique into the can design.

Anytime a new element is incorporated into the can making, thorough testing is required, the Martin Garrix black light can is no different. Through the diligence of the producer's skilled aerosol packaging reprographic team and shared learning from the producer's beverage bottle business, the technique passes all the tests without problem.

The can launched commercially in September, 2018, and to promote the partnership and product launch, Axe and Garrix released a music video that features the can(https://www.youtube.com/watch?v=DylzGXE ibU), which has garnered over 50 million views and counting.

The Axe Martin Garrix black light can is a limited edition product sold in key Latin American markets, and the partnership between Axe and Martin Garrix ladders up to a larger music platform initiative from Axe featuring many well-known and emerging artists.

To date, the producer's aerosol packaging division is the only aerosol can supplier to successfully bring this innovative can printing technique to market.

The producer and Unilever are excited to provide another innovative, sustainable packaging option to consumers.

中文介绍

6 号罐：

已上市罐

产品说明：

作为供应商,生产商为公司带来的众多优势之一是跨部门和各种金属罐的制造的知识共享。生产商的饮料事业部之前为一家大型啤酒客户开发了一种黑光光刻解决方案,基于从这个项目中吸取的经验,他们的气雾剂包装事业部开发了这种印刷技术。他们创造出一种略微进化的黑光印刷版本,并相信如果遇到合适的客户和项目,这将是一项伟大的创新。

Martin Garrix 限量版联合利华 Axe 罐登场了。Axe 与荷兰 DJ 兼制作人 Martin Garrix 的辉煌合作,为在喷雾罐上引入黑光提供了绝佳机会。这位 22 岁的艺术家最近发行了一首与 Khalid 合作的歌曲《海洋》,并曾担任全球多个大型音乐节的压轴嘉宾,甚至在韩国冬奥会闭幕式上表演。简而言之,Martin Garrix 是 Axe 完美的代言人。在联合利华的一份新闻稿中,Axe 全球副总裁 Rik Strubel 表示,"音乐似乎是 Axe 品牌的自然延伸,我们一直在追求吸引力,音乐有能力将人们聚集在一起,所以我们知道我们想在这个领域做得更多。Garrix 是年轻人的一个很好的榜样,他在这么年轻的时候就取得了这么多的成就,他拥有天生的自信,这与 Axe 的品牌相契合。我们非常荣幸地宣布他将成为 Axe 音乐的品牌大使,并期待与他一起创造出令人惊叹的作品"。

当 San Luis Potosi 的制片人团队得知这一合作关系时,他们非常热切与渴望,因为 Garrix 在墨西哥市场最为成功。他的现场演出的推广和报道描绘了一种环境,在这种环境中,Garrix 的品牌照明实际上照亮了夜晚。很明显,没有比模仿这种照明效果并将其应用于喷雾罐更好的方式来扩展他的品牌影响力了。生产商和联合利华开始合作,将生产商的黑光技术融入罐体设计中。

每当将新的元素融入罐体制造时,都需要进行彻底的测试,Martin Garrix 的黑光罐也不例外。在经验丰富的喷雾包装制版团队的勤奋努力以及从饮料瓶装业务中的学习,该技术顺利通过了所有测试。

这款罐头于 2018 年 9 月正式上市,为了推广此次合作和产品发布,Axe 和 Garrix 推出了一部以罐头为主题的音乐视频(https://www.youtube.com/watch? v = DylzGXEibU),该视频的观看次数已超过 5000 万次,且数字仍在不断攀升。

Axe Martin Garrix 黑光罐是仅在拉丁美洲为主要市场销售的限量版产品,Axe 与 Martin Garrix 的合作是 Axe 推出的一项更大音乐平台的一部分,该平台将许多知名和新兴艺术家聚集在一起。到目前为止,该生产商的喷雾包装部门是唯一一家成功将这一创新的罐体印刷技术推向市场的供应商。生产商和联合利华都对能为消费者提供另一种创新、可持续的包装选择感到兴奋。

2019-6 号罐 360 度旋转视频二维码

编号：2019-7

英文介绍

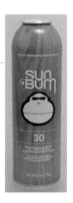

Can No. 7: Sun Bum

Marketed Can

Description: The wood effect graphics, printed with a matte over varnish provides a soft, realistic depiction in line with the Sun Bum brand.

The variation in colour from light to dark effectively communicates the product's protective qualities/sun protection factor.

中文介绍

7 号罐：

已上市罐

产品说明：

采用哑光覆膜印刷的木纹图案，与 Sun Bum 品牌相符，呈现出柔软、逼真的效果。从浅色到深色的色彩变化有效地传达了产品的保护特性/防晒指数。

2019-7 号罐 360 度旋转视频二维码

编号：2019-8

英文介绍

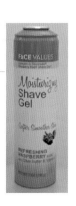

Can No. 8: Fruit of the Earth Face Values—Raspberry Shave Gel

Marketed Can

Description: This can has 7 oz, 53 mm×185 mm, featuring snaplock 4 shoulder, white base coating, dry offset printed graphics, gloss over varnish, and 2Q pressure rating. The graphics are complex due to the realistic CMYK image of the raspberry graphic supplied, and the customer wants a photographic quality reproduction. So, the producer goes to work using his proprietary dry dot screening and dry offset color separation techniques. He uses his dot gain curves to make sure the screened area in the raspberry produced to the correct final color. He also uses a split ink well to gain a soft fade of dark pink to the lighter pink color used toward the middle of the can. This item requires use of all 9-color ink stations at the litho printer and all of the graphics printed over a white base coating. The production team does an excellent job at making sure this transition is done per the customer's specifications and the screened image of the raspberry reproduced sharp and clean. Also, thanks to the digital platemaking, the producer is able to make very accurate plates and holds those screened graphics as the customer wanted.

中文介绍

8号罐：

已上市罐

产品说明：

这个罐子有7盎司重,53 mm×185 mm,采用具4个肩部的弹簧锁,白色底涂层,干胶印图案,高光油,2Q压力等级的设计。由于所提供的覆盆子图像具有逼真的四分色图像效果,因此图形比较复杂,客户希望有高品质的再现。因此,生产商开始使用自己专利的干点丝网印刷和干胶印分色技术。他使用网点增益曲线来确保覆盆子区域印出逼真的最终颜色。他还使用了一个分墨槽,以获得从较深的粉红色到较浅的粉红色的渐变效果,用于向罐子中间渐变的颜色。该产品需要在一个白色的底涂层上使用9色油墨光刻打印机打印图案。生产团队出色地完成了工作,确保覆盆子的丝网图像清晰锐利,符合客户的要求。此外,由于采用了数字制版技术,生产商能够制作出非常精确的印版,并按照客户要求保留这些丝网图案。

2019-8号罐360度旋转视频二维码

编号：2019-9

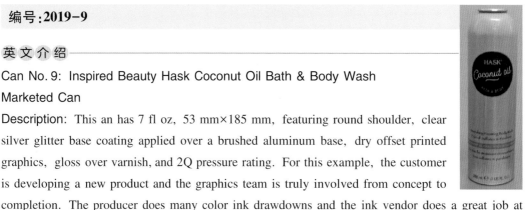

英文介绍

Can No. 9: Inspired Beauty Hask Coconut Oil Bath & Body Wash

Marketed Can

Description: This an has 7 fl oz, 53 mm×185 mm, featuring round shoulder, clear silver glitter base coating applied over a brushed aluminum base, dry offset printed graphics, gloss over varnish, and 2Q pressure rating. For this example, the customer is developing a new product and the graphics team is truly involved from concept to completion. The producer does many color ink drawdowns and the ink vendor does a great job at interpreting what was needed from the communication he had with the customer. He is developing transparent and opaque inks for this project to allow some of the brushed can marks and glitter base coat to show in some areas, but not in others. The graphics are very complex and as you can see from the printed cans the graphics team have to interpolate the final artwork for the printed cans to achieve a match the artwork supplied by the customer. He uses his dot gain curves to make sure the screened background area showing the leaf watermark pattern from top to bottom of can held open and reproduced correctly. The center blue logo on the front of the can and blue text on the back of the can are to be as opaque as possible. You'll notice a split ink well is used to help transition the transparent aqua color at the bottom of the can into an opaque white color at the top of the can. The production team does an excellent job at making sure this transition is done per the customer's specifications. Also, thanks to the producer's digital platemaking, he is able to make very accurate plates and holds those screened graphics as the customer wanted.

中文介绍

9号罐：

已上市罐

产品说明：

该罐可装7盎司,53 mm×185 mm,具有圆肩、清晰的银色闪光底涂层应用于拉丝铝基、干胶印图案、光泽的光油和2Q压力等级。客户正在开发这个新产品,而图形团队从概念到成品都真正参与其中。生产商做了很多彩色墨水的提取,而墨水供应商在解读他与客户沟通的需求方面做得很好。他正在为这个项目开发透明和不透明的墨水,以实现在某些区域显示一些刷痕和闪光底涂层,而在其他区域则不显示。图形非常复杂,正如您从印刷罐中看到的那样,图形团队必须为印刷罐插入最终的艺术品,以实现与客户提供的艺术品相匹配。他使用网点增益曲线来确保从上到下显示叶子水印图案的背景区域可以打开并正确地复制。罐子正面中心的蓝色标志和罐子背面的蓝色文字尽可能不透明。你会注意到一个分离的墨水孔被用来帮助将罐底透明的水色过渡到罐顶不透明的白色。生产团队在确保按照客户的规格完成此转换方面做得非常出色。此外,得益于制作人的数字制版,他能够完成非常精准的制版,并根据客户的需要保留那些水印图案。

2019-9号罐360度旋转视频二维码

编号：2019-10

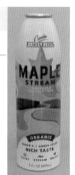

英 文 介 绍

Can No. 10: Signature Filling Coombs Family Farm Maple Stream Marketed Can

Description: This can has 7 fl oz, 53 mm×175 mm, featuring the machine curled comfort hold shoulder, white base coating, dry offset printed graphics, gloss over varnish, and 2Q pressure rating. For this example, the customer is developing a new product and the producer's graphics team is truly involved from concept to completion. The file received from the customer is a true 4-color process CMYK file with a lot of overprinting. The producer selects spot colors to help eliminate as much overprinting as possible while keeping the design as intended. The graphics are very complex and as you can see from the printed cans the graphics team have to interpolate the final artwork for the printed cans to achieve a match the artwork supplied by the customer. The proprietary color separation techniques and the dry dot screening technology uses to prevent overprinting of inks. The producer uses his dot gain curves to make sure the screened area and screened images reproduced as close to the customers artwork as possible. The production team do an excellent job at making sure this item is done per the customer specifications. Also, thanks to the digital platemaking, he is able to make very accurate plates and holds those screened graphics and tight registration as the customer wanted. They are very impressed by our capabilities during the press approval process.

中 文 介 绍

10 号罐：

已上市罐

产品说明：

　　这个罐子有 7 盎司重，53 mm×175 mm，采用机器卷边舒适握持肩部，白色底涂层，干胶印图案，高光油，2Q 压力等级的设计。例如，客户要开发一款新产品，生产商的图像团队从概念到完成都真正参与其中。但客户的文件是一个真正的 4 色印刷文件，包含大量的套印。生产商选择专色来尽可能减少套印，同时保持设计的初衷。图像非常复杂，正如您从印刷罐中看到的那样，图像团队必须为印刷罐插人最终的图片，以实现与客户提供的艺术作品的匹配。制造商使用了专有的分色技术和干网点筛选技术用于防止油墨套印。生产商使用其点扩展曲线来确保屏幕区域和屏幕图像尽可能接近客户的艺术作品。生产商在确保该产品符合客户要求方面做得非常好。此外，由于采用了数字制版技术，他们能够制作出非常精确的印版，并能够将筛网图像和精确的套准保持在客户所期望的水平。他们对我们印刷审批过程中所展现的能力印象深刻。

2019-10 号罐 360 度旋转视频二维码

编号：2019-11

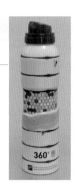

英 文 介 绍

Can No. 11: 360°

Prototypes Can

Description:

Varied shaping available around the entire circumference of the can.

Stock and proprietary shapes available.

Artwork oriented to the relief area complements the shaping.

The result of this shaping is a can that is visually engaging from every angle, while providing additional grip for usability and ergonomic effect.

Prior to 360° technology, brands are relegated to spot embossing and uniform contouring. 360° makes those restrictions a thing of the past and allows for greater customization and design opportunities.

The true beauty of the 360° technique is found where lithography and embossing intersect. Ball's 360° process ensures the artwork and relief area are aligned to further emphasize the angles and depth of shaping.

More than just a pretty designs, 360° is perfect for adding a more ergonomic grip to the package.

Though fresh off the presses, the Ball 360° sample cans have received significant early interest from major IBOs and packaging designers alike, and commercial work is in development.

The design of each sample can is thoughtfully selected for what its subject could convey about the 360° technique. The beehive can beautifully demonstrates the asymmetrical embossing capability, as well as how the added depth can play into creative, whimsical graphic designs.

Conversely, the clean lined futuristic can demonstrates the precise artwork alignment with the embossed area, and how complementary artwork can trick the eye into seeing even greater definition between the recessed area and the rest of the can.

No matter which design you prefer, there's no denying the Ball 360° cans make a statement from every angle.

中 文 介 绍

11 号罐：

样品罐

产品说明：

罐子的整个圆周上都可以进行多种图案的设计。

有库存图案和专有图案可供选择。

浮雕形的艺术图案设计使罐子从每个角度看都具有视觉吸引力，同时提供更好的抓握力，提升了适用性并更加贴合人体工程学。

在 360°技术出现之前,品牌只能进行局部浮雕和统一轮廓设计。360°技术使这些局限性成为过去,并允许进行更多的定制和设计选择。

360°技术真正的魅力在于平版印刷和浮雕的交融。Ball 的 360°工艺确保图案和浮雕区域对齐,进一步强调了造型角度和成型深度。

360°技术不仅仅是漂亮的设计,它还完美地呈现了一个更符合人体工程学的抓握感。

Ball 的 360°样品罐虽然刚刚推出,但已获得了重要的国际组织和包装设计师的浓厚兴趣,商业合作正在开发中。

每个样品罐都是经过精心设计的,以展示 360°技术所能传达的主题信息。蜂窝罐可以完美地展示不对称浮雕,通过增加深度为创意、奇特的图案设计增添趣味。

相反,线条简洁的未来主义风格罐则展示了浮雕与艺术作品之间的精确联系,以及如何通过互补的艺术作品引起视觉上的错觉,在凹陷区域与罐子其余部分之间看到更大的对比,从而产生更清晰的视觉效果。

无论你更喜欢哪种设计,都无法否认 Ball 的 360°罐子从每个角度都能展现出独特的魅力。

2019-11 号罐 360 度旋转视频二维码

编号:2019-11-1

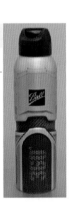

英 文 介 绍

Can No. 11-1: 360°

Prototypes Can

Description:

Varied shaping available around the entire circumference of the can.

Stock and proprietary shapes available.

Artwork oriented to the relief area complements the shaping.

The result of this shaping is a can that is visually engaging from every angle, while providing additional grip for usability and ergonomic effect.

Prior to 360° technology, brands are relegated to spot embossing and uniform contouring. 360° makes those restrictions a thing of the past and allows for greater customization and design opportunities.

The true beauty of the 360° technique is found where lithography and embossing intersect. Ball's 360° process ensures the artwork and relief area are aligned to further emphasize the angles and depth of shaping.

More than just a pretty designs, 360° is perfect for adding a more ergonomic grip to the package.

Though fresh off the presses, the Ball 360° sample cans have received significant early interest from major IBOs and packaging designers alike, and commercial work is in development.

The design of each sample can is thoughtfully selected for what its subject could convey about the 360° technique. The beehive can beautifully demonstrates the asymmetrical embossing capability, as well as how the added depth can play into creative, whimsical graphic designs.

Conversely, the clean lined futuristic can demonstrates the precise artwork alignment with the embossed area, and how complementary artwork can trick the eye into seeing even greater definition between the recessed area and the rest of the can.

No matter which design you prefer, there's no denying the Ball 360° cans make a statement from every angle.

中 文 介 绍

11-1 号罐:

样品罐

产品说明:

罐子的整个圆周上都可以进行多种图案的设计。

有库存图案和专有图案可供选择。

浮雕形的艺术图案设计使罐子从每个角度看都具有视觉吸引力,同时提供更好的抓握力,提升了适用性并更加贴合人体工程学。

在 360°技术出现之前,品牌只能进行局部浮雕和统一轮廓设计。360°技术使这些局限性成为过去,并允许进行更多的定制和设计选择。

360°技术真正的魅力在于平版印刷和浮雕的交融。Ball 的 360°工艺确保图案和浮雕区域对齐,进一步强调了造型角度和成型深度。

360°技术不仅仅是漂亮的设计,它还完美地呈现了一个更符合人体工程学的抓握感。

Ball 的 360°样品罐虽然刚刚推出,但已获得了重要的国际组织和包装设计师的浓厚兴趣,商业合作正在开发中。

每个样品罐都是经过精心设计的,以展示 360°技术所能传达的主题信息。蜂窝罐可以完美地展示不对称浮雕,通过增加深度为创意、奇特的图案设计增添趣味。

相反,线条简洁的未来主义风格罐则展示了浮雕与艺术作品之间的精确联系,以及如何通过互补的艺术作品引起视觉上的错觉,在凹陷区域与罐子其余部分之间看到更大的对比,从而产生更清晰的视觉效果。

无论你更喜欢哪种设计,都无法否认 Ball 的 360°罐子从每个角度都能展现出独特的魅力。

2019-11-1 号罐 360 度旋转视频二维码

七、2018 年国际铝气雾罐竞赛参赛罐

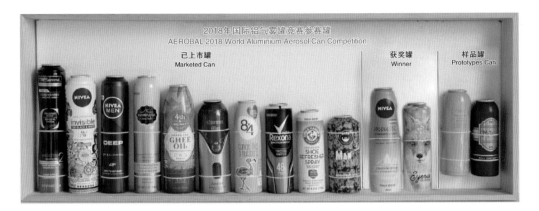

罐编号从左至右分别是:14,2,5,6,7,11,1,4,8,10,3,13,9,12

编号:2018-1

英 文 介 绍

Can No. 1: Beiersdorf 8×4—Limited Edition

Marketed Can

Description: A new fresh appearance of the famous 8×4 brand.

The cans are perfect examples how a brand known since 1951 can be appealing to a younger generation in 2018. The printing shows a modern design that appeals to teenagers and young at heart. Each design has its own personal message not only visible by words but also through the artwork. The cans have got an innovative print-barely visible to the naked eye. The background is made up of two different colours out of the same colour spectrum. They softly fade into each other and meet in the lower half of the can. The clear naive art complements the background. On average, an artwork is made up of 6-8 colours. The new 8×4 range includes designs printed with up to 10 colours, realized through ink tray separation. The whole can/range carries the spirit of the times (zeitgeist).

中 文 介 绍

1 号罐:

已上市罐

产品说明:

这是著名的 8×4 商标的全新外观。

这些罐体是 1951 年以来就为人所知的品牌如何在 2018 年吸引年轻一代的完美范例。其

印刷图案是具有吸引青少年和童心未泯的年轻人的现代设计。每个设计都有其专属信息,不仅表现在文字中,还表现在图案中。罐体上有一些肉眼几乎看不见的创新的图案。其背景由同一色谱的两种不同颜色组成。这两种颜色在罐体的下半部分柔和地融入彼此。清晰朴素的艺术图案与背景相得益彰。一般来说,一件艺术品由 6~8 种颜色组成。新的 8×4 系列包括多达 10 种颜色的印刷设计,通过墨盘分离实现。整个罐子系列产品都体现了时代精神。

2018-1 号罐 360 度旋转视频二维码

编号:**2018-2**

英文介绍

Can No. 2: Invisible for Black & White Limited Edition by Matthew Williamson for BDF Nivea

Marketed Can

Description: An outstanding ornamental print design in mostly black and white. Colour is added by blooms and butterflies. The contrast of blooms and butterflies compared to the clear lines and borders makes this print design so unique and lively. The extremely detailed borders appear even at the very base of the can but also between the text on the back side of the can, which makes a pleasant change. Even the description of the closure is surrounded by ornaments and a butterfly, which is very unusual. The print shows an overall perfect preference for detail. This can looks like a piece of art.

中文介绍

2 号罐:

已上市罐

产品说明:

这是一款以黑白为主色调的精美图案设计。通过花朵和蝴蝶增添了色彩,与清晰的线条和边框的对比使这款印刷设计更加独特而生动。极其细致的边框既出现在罐子底部,也出现在罐子背面的文字之间,这让人耳目一新。甚至连罐体的封盖也被装饰和蝴蝶包围,看起来不同凡响。这款印刷设计作品展示了对细节的整体完美偏好,看起来就像一件艺术品。

2018-2 号罐 360 度旋转视频二维码

编号:2018-3

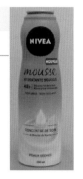

英 文 介 绍

Can No. 3: Nivea Body Mousse

Marketed Can

Description: The Nivea Body Mousse is developed exclusively for aerosol application. This mousse is smooth and light, like a white fluffy cloud and is easy to dispense. The shape of the can ensures that the can fits perfectly in one's hand. This can is the ultimate combination of content, shape and print. The can displays an outstanding smooth conical shape. Creating such a shape requires a great deal of attention to the details.

Shaping:

Production tooling for the Nivea mousse can is done with "spline technology". This technology is used to achieve a smooth and fine transition on the shape and to avoid shadowing on the can surface. The stepped shoulder, specially adapted to the spray cap geometry, requires shaping in small steps. Everything from drawing to tool setting has to be precisely aligned in order to get to a perfect can.

Printing:

Pre-press work is required to modify the brand logo in such a way that after shaping, the logo looks perfectly round on the final can. In the first place, when printed onto the cylindrical can, the logo is totally unregularly pre-distorted. It is then shaped horizontally and vertically—which makes it even more difficult to evaluate in which way it has to be designed before shaping. The very fine and seamless colour graduation from an opaque violet running down from the top to the base of the can into a pale violet, is outstanding. The mousse and the white drop of Karite butter owe their real look to the subtle screens used in the printing process. You can more or less feel the softness and smoothness of the mousse.

中 文 介 绍

3号罐:

已上市罐

产品说明:

妮维雅身体摩丝是专为喷雾应用而开发的。这款摩丝质地轻盈细腻,如一朵洁白的蓬松云朵,易于使用。罐子的形状确保其完美贴合手掌。这款罐子是内容、形状和印刷的完美结合。罐子呈现出非常光滑的圆锥形。创造出这样的形状需要对细节精心处理。

成型:妮维雅摩丝罐的生产模具采用"样条技术"。这种技术用于实现形状的平滑精细过渡,避免罐体表面出现阴影。特别设计的阶梯式肩部需要分步成型。为了获得完美的罐体,从绘图到模具设置的每一个步骤都需要精确一致。

印刷:印刷前需要修改品牌标志,使其定型后在最终罐子上看起来非常完美。首先,将品牌标志印刷在圆柱形罐子上时,它是完全不规则且失真的,需要在水平方向和垂直方向上进行塑形——这使得在塑形之前更难以评估以何种方式设计。从顶部到底部,罐子的颜色从不透明的紫色到淡紫色,这种精密无缝的色彩渐变效果令人瞩目。印刷过程中使用细微网版,使摩丝和白色的卡利特黄油滴看起来非常逼真。让人或多或少感受到摩丝的柔软和顺滑。

2018-3 号罐 360 度旋转视频二维码

编号:2018-4

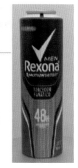

英文介绍

Can No. 4: Rexona Limited Edition

Marketed Can

Description: A masculine can for the South American soccer fan. The buyer can choose its favourite team as the colours resemble some of the soccer teams national soccer jersey for the upcoming Soccer World Championship. The combination of o-paque and translucent print makes the artwork interesting. Different stages of opacity are used on this can. The opaque black is achieved by using a second hit with black. The brand logo and writing is done in negative print and shows the brushed aluminium. In contrast the centrepiece is a translucent colour where the brushed aluminium shines through and gives this colour a metallic look.

中文介绍

4 号罐:

已上市罐

产品说明:

　　这是一款专为南美足球迷设计的带有阳刚之美的罐子。买家可以选择自己喜欢的球队,因为罐子的颜色与即将到来的世界杯足球赛的一些国家队球衣颜色相似。半透明和不透明的印刷图案的结合使其更加有趣。罐体上运用了不同程度的不透明度设计。其中不透明的黑色是通过黑色的双版套印来实现的。品牌标志和文字采用透底技术,显示出磨砂铝的质感。与此形成对比的是,中心部分是半透明色,磨砂铝的光泽闪闪发光,呈现出金属质感。

2018-4 号罐 360 度旋转视频二维码

编号：2018-5

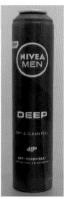

Can No. 5: Nivea Deep Black

Marketed Can

Description: A cool masculine can. The carbon design is printed with dark grey and black to perfection (perfect registration) and is an eye-catcher. The can displays actually two different types of black which are divided by an even deeper black gradient. To achieve the deep black the colour is applied twice to ensure a high opacity. The can is brushed and the front side letters are printed in perfect negative print to show off the brushed aluminium. The brand logo is surrounded by a very thin black line to ensure the perfect round shape of the NIVEA Logo.

中 文 介 绍

5 号罐：

已上市罐

产品说明：

这是一款酷炫的男性香水罐。采用深灰色和黑色完美对齐的碳素设计印刷,非常引人注目。它实际上展示了两种不同的黑色,它们被一个更深的渐变黑色隔开。为了达到深黑色的效果,印了两遍黑色,以确保图案的高不透明度。罐子经过上漆,其正面的字母采用透底印刷,以突出抛光铝的质感。品牌标志被一条非常细的黑线环绕,以确保妮维雅标志的完美圆形形状。

2018-5 号罐 360 度旋转视频二维码

编号：2018-6

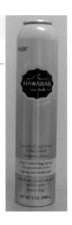

Can No. 6: KIK Hask Hawaiian Dry Texturizing Spray

Marketed Can

Description: This can has 5 floz, 45 mm×190 mm, round shoulder, brushed can with silver glitter base coating, dry offset printed graphics, gloss over varnish, 2Q pressure rating and PAM interior coating. For this example, the customer is developing a new product and our graphics team is truly involved from concept to completion. We do many colour ink drawdowns and our ink vendor do a great job at interpreting what is needed from the communication we have with the customer. We are developing transparent and opaque inks for this project to allow some of the brushed can marks and glitter base coat to show in some areas but not in others. The graphics are very complex and as you can see from the printed cans our graphics team have to interpolate the final artwork for the printed cans to achieve a match the artwork supplied by the customer. We use our dot gain curves to make sure the screened area around the front panel logo showing the flowers and leave pattern held open and re-produced correctly. Finally, you'll notice a split ink well used to transition the transparent aqua colour at the bottom of the can into an opaque white colour at the top of the can. Our production team do an excellent job at making sure this transition is done per the customer specifications. Also, thanks to our digital platemaking, we are able to make very accurate plates and hold those screened graphics as the customer wanted.

中文介绍

6 号罐：

已上市罐

产品说明：

该罐重 5 盎司,尺寸为 45 mm×190 mm,圆肩设计,表面采用银色闪光底涂层,干式胶印图案,刷高光光油,2Q 压力等级和 PAM 内涂层。例如,这个例子中,客户正在开发一款新产品,我们的设计团队从概念到完成都全程参与。我们做了很多颜色的油墨试样,油墨供应商在理解我们与客户沟通的需求方面做得非常好。我们正在为这个项目开发透明和不透明的油墨,以便让刷漆罐的痕迹和银色底涂层在某些区域显示出来,而在其他区域则不显示。这些图案非常复杂,从印刷罐上的印刷图案可以看出,我们的图形设计团队必须在有油墨的罐上插入最终的图案,确保与客户提供的图案一致。我们使用网点增益曲线来确保前罐子面板上的花卉和叶子图案周围的印刷区域保持开放状态并正确再现。最后,您会注意到一个分墨槽,用于将罐底的透明的水绿色转换为罐顶的不透明白色。我们的制作团队在确保按客户要求完成转换方面做得非常出色。此外,由于我们采用数字制版技术,我们可以制作出非常精准的印版,并按照客户要求保存这些网屏图像。

2018-6 号罐 360 度旋转视频二维码

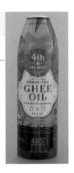

编号：2018-7

英文介绍

Can No. 7: Signature Filling 4th & Heart Ghee Oil

Marketed Can

Description: This can has 5 floz, 53 mm×175 mm, comfort shoulder, white base coating, dry offset printed graphics, gloss over varnish, 2Q pressure rating and epoxy-phenolic interior coating. The challenges are many fold. Our customer provides a sample done previously using shrink sleeved technology. The graphics are very complex and as you can see from the printed cans we need all (9) ink stations and this job has to be completed with super accurate registration. Our graphics group have to interpolate the final artwork for the printed cans to match the artwork and visual appearance of the previously printed sample. The tropical scene reproduction is a challenge for sure. We complete many colour matches trying to achieve the colour matches as done on the shrink sleeve. Finally, if you zoom in on the engraved leaf pattern at the bottom of the can you will see the very fine details of that reproduction. This area is much more defined than our sample provided with the shrink sleeve. Some of these lines are very thin at only about (0.003-5″) thickness and thanks to our digital platemaking we are able to make very accurate plates and hold those thin lines as the customer wanted. Our production staff do an excellent job in matching the graphics to the proof we provided.

中文介绍

7 号罐：

已上市罐

产品说明：

该罐有 5 盎司重,53 mm×175 mm,舒适的肩型设计、白色底涂层、干式胶印图案、过高光油、2Q 压力等级和环氧酚醛内部涂层。挑战是多方面的。我们的客户提供了以前使用的收缩套管技术制作的样品,样品的图案非常复杂。从印刷的罐子上可以看到,我们需要所有(9 个)色彩的油墨,这项工作必须以超高的精确度来完成。我们的图案组团队必须在有油墨的罐子上插入最终的图案,使得与先前印刷样品的图案和视觉外观保持一致。热带场景的再现无疑是一个挑战。我们尝试了多种颜色匹配,从而达到与收缩套管上的颜色一致。最后,如果你放大罐子底部雕刻的叶子图案,你会看到复制的细节非常精细。这个区域比我们提供的带有收缩膜的样本要精细得多。其中一些线条非常细,只有大约 0.003—5 英寸的厚度,多亏了我们的数字制版技术,我们能够制作出非常精确的印版,并根据客户的需要保留这些细线。我们的制作团队在将图像与我们提供的样稿相匹配方面做得非常出色。

2018-7 号罐 360 度旋转视频二维码

编号：2018-8

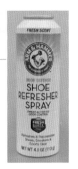

英 文 介 绍

Can No. 8: American Spraytech Arm & Hammer Shoe Refresher Marketed Can

Description: This can has 4.0 floz, 45 mm×135 mm, flat 45 shoulder, white base coating, dry offset printed graphics, gloss over varnish, 2Q pressure rating and PAM interior coating. The graphics are complex due to the Arm & Hammer trademark glow rays or starburst patterns extended from the Arm & Hammer red circular logo on the front and back panels. We rework the customer file to give us a soft transition from positive dot to reverse dot in the screening pattern. The red halftone image of the trademarked arm is also very important and as you can see from the printed cans our graphics team have to interpolate the final artwork for the printed cans to achieve a match the artwork supplied by the customer. We use our dot gain curves to make sure the screened area in the arm produced the correct final colour. Finally, you'll notice a split ink well used to transition the orange colour at the top of the can from 100% to 0 at the midway point of the can. Our production team do an excellent job at making sure this transition is done per the customer specifications. Also, thanks to our digital platemaking, we are able to make very accurate plates and hold those screened graphics as the customer wanted.

中 文 介 绍

8 号罐：

已上市罐

产品说明：

该罐可装 4.0 盎司,45 mm×135 mm,平肩 45 度、白色底涂层、干胶印图案、过光油、2Q 压力等级以及 PAM 内涂层。由于 Arm & Hammer 商标的光芒射线或星形图案从其红色圆形标志延伸到前后面上,导致图案非常复杂。我们重新处理了客户文件,以在加网图案中提供从正点到反点的平滑过渡。正如你从印刷罐中看到的那样,商标上部的红色半色调图像非常重要,我们的图案团队必须为印刷罐插入最终的图案,以实现与客户提供的图案相一致。我们使用网点增益曲线来确保商标上部的筛选区域最终产生正确的颜色。最后,你会注意到有一条分墨槽,它可以将橙色从罐体顶部的 100% 过渡到罐子中间的 0。我们的制作团队在确保按照客户的期望完成这个转换方面做得非常出色。此外,多亏了我们的数字制版技术,我们能够完成非常精准的制版,并根据客户的需要保留那些屏幕图案。

2018-8 号罐 360 度旋转视频二维码

编号：2018-9

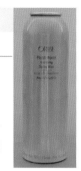

Can No. 9: Oribe Flash Form Finishing Spray

Prototypes Can

Description: Wax 150mL 45 mm×140 mm, oval shoulder, brushed surface and gold transparent base coating, dry offset printed graphics, gloss over varnish, 2Q pressure rating, and epoxy-phenolic interior coating. The challenges are many fold. Our customer provide a mock-up sample created by their modelling agency for visual colour and graphic reproduction and used in their marketing materials. Our graphics group have to interpolate the final artwork for the printed cans to match the artwork and visual appearance of the mock-up sample. The customer provide a sample plastic jar with gold foil hot stamping and they want the cashmere colour of the background colour of the aerosol can to match the colour of the plastic jar. We do many colour matches, and finally settled on overprinting the cashmere colour over the gold base coating. This helps to achieve the richness and depth of colour with more opaqueness like the plastic jar provided. The application of the gold base coating is also a challenge since the customer wanted that foil hot stamp look. Finally, if you zoom in on the vertical lines of the graphics reversed out of the background colour, you'll see very thin lines of black key lines highlighting the vertical lines. These are very thin at only about 0.003″ thickness and thanks to our digital plate-making we are able to make very accurate plates and hold those thin lines as the customer wanted. We use a double hit plate technique to also make sure the density of the cashmere coloured ink for the background colour is very dense and covered the brushed metal of the can as much as possible. Our production staff do an excellent job in communication between the customer and their designer who both are on site for the press approval. Overall our customer is very happy with the final results and this new product launch has been a very big success.

9 号罐：

样品罐

产品说明：

该罐可装蜂蜡 150 mL，45 mm×140 mm，具有椭圆形肩、抛光表面和金色透明底涂层、干胶印刷、高光油、2Q 压力等级以及环氧酚醛内涂层。挑战是多方面的。我们的客户提供了一个由他们的模型机构制作的样本，用于视觉效果和图案复制，并用于他们的营销材料。我们的图案组必须在油墨罐子上插入最终的图案，以使图案和模型样本的视觉外观保持一致。客户提供了一个用金箔烫印的塑料罐样品，他们希望气雾剂罐的金色底色与塑料罐的颜色相匹配。我们做了很多颜色的匹配，最终决定在金色的底涂层上套印丝光颜色。这有助于实现类似于塑料罐提供的更柔和的深色调和丰富的色彩。金色底涂层的应用也是一个挑战，因为客户想要获得烫金效果。最后，如果你放大与背景颜色相反的图形的竖线，你会看到非常细的黑线突出了竖线。这些线条非常薄,只有大约 0.003 英寸。多亏我们的数字制版,我们能够制作出非常精准的制版,并根据客户的需要保留这些细线。我们使用了双套印技术,确保作为背景色的丝光彩色油墨的密度非常密集,并尽可能地覆盖了抛光拉丝金属。我们的生产人员在客户和他们的设计师之间的沟通方面做得很好,他们都在现场参与了印刷审批。总的来说,我们的客户对最终结果非常满意,这次新产品的推出取得了巨大的成功。

2018-9 号罐 360 度旋转视频二维码

编号:2018-10

英文介绍

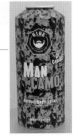

Can No. 10: GIBS Man Camo Aerosol Body Spray Go Fresh
Marketed Can

Description: Fort Collins based GIBS Grooming, recently introduced its first-ever body spray, just in time for summer. Man camo aerosol body spray lands in a crisp, clean go coastal scent, ideal for summer smell-good on the go. The container for this strapping fragrance is a distinctive, highly decorated conical shoulder aluminum aerosol can. The graphics utilize various colours and with kiss fit registration, the producer is able to replicate digital camouflage for this contemporary concept. Trendy, matte over varnish is the obvious choice as the finishing touch to enhance this rugged design. The masculine appearance is created to capture the customers attention, while the superfine spray refreshes the flesh with crisp, clean hints of driftwood, sea salt, citrus, patchouli and musk.

中文介绍

10 号罐:

已上市罐

产品说明:

总部位于柯林斯堡的 GIBS 美容公司最近推出了首款身体喷雾剂,恰逢夏季来临。名为“Man camo”的男士迷彩喷雾式身体香水喷雾散发出清新的海岸气味,是夏季出行时保持良好气味的理想选择。这个包装香水的容器是一只独特的、装饰精美的圆锥形铝制气雾剂罐。罐体表面使用了多种颜色,并带有轻浮于其中的图案,生产商能够用现代概念的产品复制这些数码迷彩图案。时尚的哑光光油作为设计的点睛之笔,增强了这款粗犷设计的质感。这款男性化的设计旨在吸引顾客的注意,而超细喷雾则能为肌肤带来清新、干净的木屑、海盐、柑橘、薄荷和麝香的香味。

2018-10 号罐 360 度旋转视频二维码

编号：2018-11

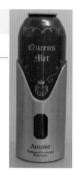

英文介绍

Can No. 11: QUEENS MET-Ametist

Marketed Can

Description: The shape of the can is named "El Fantastico". With its 360 degrees oriented-printed deformation & deep shaping down to 90 mm from thé can top, the can is a real-value added significantly distinctive product. Aside from its unique oriental shape and lively gold colours, it has an oriental gold-plated glossy cap, which resembles the elegancy of a queen, just like the new brand. The brand "Queens Met" has recently been launched by Sora Cosmetics, Turkey, one of the major clients of the producer, who is expanding their various brands in the Middle East region as well as North Africa.

The brand is well-protected against product counterfeiting owing to the oriented printed deformation which had been launched by the producer a couple of years ago.

中文介绍

11 号罐：

已上市罐

产品说明：

这个罐的形状被命名为"E! Fantastico"。该罐具有 360 度可变形定向印刷以及从罐顶向下 90 mm 的深度成型，是一款真正具有显著附加值的独特产品。除了具有东方特色的造型和耀眼的金色外观外，它还有一个具有东方特色的镀金的光亮盖子，与新品牌的优雅相得益彰。"Queens Met"品牌由土耳其主要客户之一 Sora Cosmetics 推出，该公司正在中东地区以及北非拓展其各种品牌。由于生产商几年前推出了定向印刷变形技术，该品牌在防止产品假冒方面具有很好的保护作用。

2018-11 号罐 360 度旋转视频二维码

编号：**2018-12**

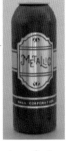

英 文 介 绍

Can No. 12: Metallic Rise and Shine Can

Prototypes Can

Description: There's just something about shiny objects. That metallic glimmer catches your eye and draws you to the shelf. Gleaming like a diamond, reflecting extravagance, excellence and beauty. The producer's metallic ink creates a distinct, premium feel.

For years, many customers gravitated toward the producer's hot stamping technique (where a metallic foil is applied to the can) but hot stamping can be a price prohibitive design option. With budget an understandable concern the producer explores techniques using metallic inks to achieve a comparable rich, brilliant effect that will provide a more affordable, but equally enchanting solution. Using state of the art pigments and the producer's unique ink application technology, a glossy, reflective sheen is achievable in a range of metallic shades. The producer is able to apply their metallic technique on aluminium cans of all shapes and sizes. Too often innovation happens in isolation, but the producer firmly believes in co-innovation and considers the market's needs when prioritizing innovation initiatives. After countless inquiries about hot stamping then customers pulling back from the price, it becomes clear that the aesthetic of something highly reflective and glossy is desired on the shelf. This can is designed to have an intentional French apothecary feel with a modern twist. Given that most of the market is familiar with seeing hot stamping on more luxury cans such as perfumes or high-end body sprays, the producer sought a design that could go head-to-head with hot stamping. Achieving a finish on an aluminium aerosol can that rivals hot stamping is not an easy reprographic feat and took quite a bit of R & D to achieve the desired effect. The producer developed a unique ink and coating application technology which is combined with matte and gloss process. In the past silver inks have tended to look grey or matte and therefore have not given the sheen that is comparable to a hot stamp. However, using the producer's proprietary process gives the silver a mirror-like finish that is desirable to the customer for a variety of brands.

中 文 介 绍

12 号罐：

样品罐

产品说明：

闪亮的物体总有一种魔力。金属的光泽吸引着你的目光,将你引向货架。它像钻石一样闪耀,展现着奢华、卓越和美丽。制造商的金属油墨创造出一种独特的高级感。多年来,许多客户被生产商的烫印技术(在罐上烫印金属箔),但烫印可能是一种价格昂贵的设计选择。考虑到预算问题,生产商探索了使用金属油墨的技术,以实现与烫印同样丰富、明亮的效果,从而提供更经济实惠、同样迷人的解决方案。使用最先进的颜料和生产商独特的油墨应用技术,可以实现一系列金属色调的光泽、反射效果。生产商能够在各种形状和尺寸的铝罐上应用其金属油墨技术。太多时候,创新是孤立的,但生产商坚信协同创新,在优先考虑创新举措时要考虑市场的需求。在对烫印进行了无数次的询问后,客户又因价格问题而退缩,这表明消费者渴望在货架上看到高反光的和有光泽的很有美感的外观。这款罐子的设计旨在有意营造出法国药房的感觉,同时带有现代风格。鉴于大多数市场都很常见在香水或高端身体喷雾等更奢华的罐子上使用烫印,因此生产商寻求一种能够与烫印相抗衡的设计。在铝制喷雾罐上实现与烫印相媲美的效果并不是一项容易的技术,需要进行大量的研发以达到预期效果。生产商开发了一种独特的油墨和涂层应用技术,结合了哑光和亮光工艺。过去,银色油墨往往看起来是灰色或哑光的,因此无法与烫印的光泽相媲美。然而,使用生产商的专有工艺可以使银色具有镜面般的光泽,这是各种品牌的消费者所渴望的。

2018-12 号罐 360 度旋转视频二维码

编号:2018-13

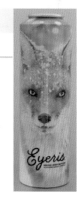

英文介绍

Can No. 13: Eyeris Fox Can

Prototypes Can

Description: Historically, aluminium aerosol customers have had to shy away from imagery for their brand with graphics containing photo-realistic human skin, or detail and varied textures, such as floral prints, fruit, vegetables, animal fur, etc., because these graphics don't translate well to cans printed in the round (offset printing). The producer sees this limitation in the market as an opportunity to provide customers with a unique solution.

Eyeris was originally developed by the producer's beverage group, and so is able to leverage their learning, then adapt and enhance the technique for aluminium aerosol cans. Eyeris provides unparalleled precision that provides a 360°degree billboard for graphics that do not shy away from lifelike detail. For customers craving detailed graphics to bring their brand to life, Eyeris high definition printing is the best alternative to digital. Not only does it provide the offset printing platform so vital for bold colours, it also removes the need for expensive capital investment.

Eyeris is achieved using a proprietary technique of artwork separation and plate manufacturing which allows for 150-200 dots per inch (DPI) compared to 133 DPl for conventional printing. The commercial Eyeris process uses up to 9 colours. The Eyeris Fox Can is the second iteration of the Eyeris printing technique.

In 2018, it became evident that the producer would not only be able to provide customers with next-level execution of Eyeris but provide them with the innovation globally (previously available only in certain regions). When considering design schematics for the can we want an image that showcased the detail previously unavailable on aluminium and also something that would stand apart from other brands on the shelf. The Eyeris Fox Can exemplifies both.

中 文 介 绍

13 号罐：

样品罐

产品说明：

　　历史上,铝制喷雾剂客户一直不愿在其品牌的图形设计中使用具有照片般逼真人皮肤、细节丰富且纹理多样的图形,如花卉印花、水果、蔬菜、动物皮毛等,因为这些图形在圆形罐子(胶印)上印刷的效果不佳。生产商将这一局限性视为向客户提供独特解决方案的机会。

　　Eyeris 最初是由生产商的饮料部门开发的,因此能够利用其经验,为铝制喷雾罐改进和提升这一技术。Eyeris 提供了无与伦比的精确度,为图形提供了 360 度的全方位展示,使它们不再回避逼真的细节。对于渴望使用精致的图案设计来使品牌栩栩如生的客户来说,Eyeris 高清印刷是数字印刷的最佳替代品。它不仅提供了对鲜艳色彩至关重要的胶印平台,而且还消除了对昂贵成本的投资。Eyeris 是通过一种专有的图案分离和制版技术,它允许每英寸 150—200 个点(DPI),而传统印刷的 DPI 为 133 点。商用 Eyeris 工艺使用多达 9 种颜色。Eyeris Fox Can 是 Eyeris 印刷技术的第二代产品。

　　2018 年,生产商不仅能够为客户提供更高水平的 Eyeris 方案,还能在全球范围内提供创新(此前仅在某些地区可用)。在考虑罐体的设计草图时,我们想要一个既能展示以前在铝制材料上无法看到的细节,同时也想要设计出在货架上能够脱颖而出的东西。Eyeris Fox Can 则两者兼具。

2018-13 号罐 360 度旋转视频二维码

编号：**2018-14**

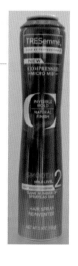

英 文 介 绍

Can No. 14: TRESemmé Hair Spray

Marketed Can

Description: Unilever approaches the producer to help develop a sustainable, innovative, full body shaped package to hold their newly formulated lines of hair sprays. With all the choices on the market today, especially at a drug store level, brands need a distinct shape that will set them apart from the competition. The package's unique design allows their product to stand out on the shelf and grab the consumer's attention. Additionally, consumers not only want a product that looks and feels good, but one that also benefits the environment. This package is 99.7% pure aluminium, making it 100% recyclable. This product is a great example of how two innovative companies can come together to produce a fully unique hair care product.

中 文 介 绍

14 号罐:

已上市罐

产品说明:

联合利华与生产商合作,开发了一种可持续创新的全方位包装,用于盛装其新研发的喷雾系列产品。如今市场上有众多选择,尤其是在药店层面的品牌,需要一种独特的形状来使自己与竞争对手区分开来。该包装独特的设计使其产品在货架上脱颖而出,吸引消费者的注意。此外,消费者不仅想要外观和手感良好的产品,还想要对环境有益的产品。这款包装是 99.7%的纯铝制成的,100%可回收。这款产品是两家创新型公司携手合作,创造出一款独一无二的护发产品的绝佳例证。

2018-14 号罐 360 度旋转视频二维码

八、2017年国际铝气雾罐竞赛参赛罐

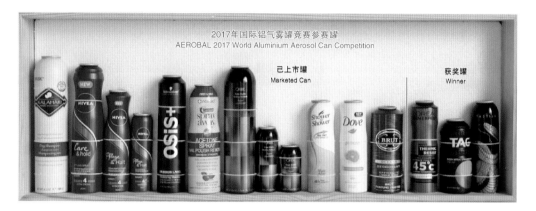

罐编号从左至右分别是:7,4a,4b,4c,12,6,5a,5b,5c,18,10,3,13,8,15

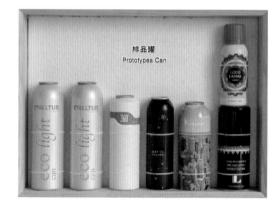

罐编号从左至右分别是:1,2,14,16,9,17

编号:2017-1

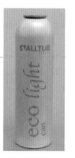

英文介绍

Can No. 1: Eco Light Can 15 bar

Prototypes Can

Description: This Can has 53 mm×173 mm, 1″ opening, ogival shoulder, 15 bar.

Innovative factor: Among the initiatives dedicated to the reduction of the environmental impact of its own products, the producer has realised an experimentation aiming to reduce the quantity of aluminium needed to produce its own cans.

The producer's goal is to research, inside its own know-how and production process, the elements that can brings as a result to a finished can with a considerably lower weight than a standard aerosol can. For such project the producer has kept its usual supply sources, no external suppliers have been involved, no innovative raw materials and tools have been experienced. Just by working with the means available to its own control, the producer has tested some variations to its own process parameters and tools which have brought to the creation of this can: Aluminium EN-3102, Deformation > 15 bar, Burst out > 18 bar, Average weight of the cans 32.4 g.

中 文 介 绍

1号罐：

样品罐

产品说明：

　　该罐53 mm×173 mm，1英寸口径，椭圆形肩部，可承受压力为15 bar（压力单位）。

　　创新因素：制造商为了减少其产品对环境的影响，实施了一些措施，其中包括一项旨在减少生产其罐子所需原料铝用量的实验。

　　制造商的目标是在自己的专业知识和生产过程中，探索找出使成品罐的重量比标准气雾罐轻得多的方法。为此，制造商既没有改变外部供应商，也没有使用任何新的原材料和工具。仅通过可控的手段，生产商对自己的工艺参数和工具进行了一些调整，最终制造出了这款铝罐：铝材EN-3102，承压大于15 bar，抗爆大于18 bar，平均重量为32.4克。

2017-1号罐360度旋转视频二维码

编号：2017-2

英 文 介 绍

Can No. 2: Eco Light Can 12 bar

Prototypes Can

Description: This can has 53 mm×173 mm, 1″ opening, ogival shoulder, 12 bar.

Innovative factor: Among the initiatives dedicated to the reduction of the environmental impact of its own products, the producer has realised an experimentation aiming to reduce the quantity of aluminium needed to produce its own cans. The producer's goal is to research, inside its own know-how and production process, the elements that can brings as a result to a finished can with a considerably lower weight than a standard aerosol can. For such project the producer has kept its usual supply sources, no external suppliers have been involved, no innovative raw materials and tools have been experienced. Just by working with the means available to its own control, the producer has tested some variations to its own process parameters and tools which have brought to the creation of this can: Aluminium EN-3102, Deformation > 12.5 bar, Burst out > 14.4 bar, verage weight of the cans 30.7 g.

中文介绍

2 号罐：

样品罐

产品说明：

该罐 53 mm×173 mm，1 英寸口径，椭圆形肩部，可承受 12 bar 压力。

创新因素：制造商为了减少其产品对环境的影响，实施了一些措施，其中包括一项旨在减少生产其罐子所需原料铝用量的实验。

制造商的目标是在自己的专业知识和生产过程中，探索找出使成品罐的重量比标准气雾罐轻得多的方法。为此，制造商既没有改变外部供应商，也没有使用任何新的原材料和工具。仅通过可控的手段，生产商对自己的工艺参数和工具进行了一些调整，最终制造出了这款铝罐：铝材 EN-3102，承压大于 12.5 bar，抗爆大于 14.4 bar，平均重量为 30.7 克。

2017-2 号罐 360 度旋转视频二维码

编号：**2017-3**

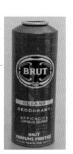

英文介绍

Can No.3: BRUT

Marketed Can

Description: A beautiful and straight forward design. The special property of this can is not visible to the eye. It is manufactured with an environmental friendly water based over varnish. Water based varnishes have been available since quite a long time—however, for limited use only. Especially the effect of the over varnish turning yellow during the drying process was a problem in the past. With this new development the issue has been fixed. The technical properties (distribution, brilliance and yellowing) are now comparable to the standard solvent based varnishes. This varnish is a step further to a more sustainable production of aluminum aerosol cans—40% of solvents are replaced by water.

中文介绍

3 号罐：

已上市罐

产品说明：

这是一款漂亮而简洁的设计。这款罐的特别之处并不明显。它采用环保型水性光油制造。之前水性光油已经出现很长一段时间了,但仅限于有限的用途。尤其是上光油在干燥过程中变黄的问题在过去一直是一个难题。有了这项新技术,这个问题迎刃而解。这种上光油的技术性能、光泽度和变黄程度现在可与标准溶剂型上光油相媲美。但它的溶剂用量减少了40%,使铝气雾罐可持续生产比之前又进了一步。

2017-3 号罐 360 度旋转视频二维码

编号:2017-4a

英文介绍

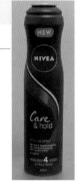

Can No. 4a: BDF Care & Hold

Marketed Can

Description: This is a series of cans in different formats. The center-piece shows a soft curl of hair. The brushed aluminum shines through the blue curl and gives the design a touch of pearle scence. The extremly fine gradation is blending into the blue background colour which contrasts the shiny centre-piece. This perfect gradation is achieved by the use of a new polymerisation technology for printing plates. The combination of the polymerization technology and laser cut printing plates makes this design so unique.

中文介绍

4a 号罐:

已上市罐

产品说明:

这是一系列不同形状的罐子。罐体中心图案展示了一头柔软的卷发。经过抛光的铝制表面在蓝色卷发的映衬下闪闪发光,为设计增添了一抹珍珠般的光泽。极其细腻的渐变色完美地融入蓝色背景中,与闪亮的中心部分形成对比。这种完美的渐变效果是通过使用一种新的印版聚合工艺技术实现的。聚合技术与激光雕刻印版技术的结合使这个设计很独特。

2017-4a 号罐 360 度旋转视频二维码

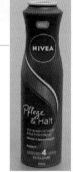

编号：2017-4b

英 文 介 绍

Can No. 4b: BDF Care & Hold (Nos. 4 a to c)

Marketed Can

Description: This is a series of cans in different formats. The center-piece shows a soft curl of hair. The brushed aluminum shines through the blue curl and gives the design a touch of pearle scence. The extremly fine gradation is blending into the blue background colour which contrasts the shiny centre-piece. This perfect gradation is achieved by the use of a new polymerisation technology for printing plates. The combination of the polymerization technology and laser cut printing plates makes this design so unique.

中 文 介 绍

4b 号罐：

已上市罐

产品说明：

这是一系列不同形状的罐子。罐体中心图案展示了一头柔软的卷发。经过抛光的铝制表面在蓝色卷发的映衬下闪闪发光，为设计增添了一抹珍珠般的光泽。极其细腻的渐变色完美地融入蓝色背景中，与闪亮的中心部分形成对比。这种完美的渐变效果是通过使用一种新的印版聚合工艺技术实现的。聚合技术与激光雕刻印版技术的结合使这个设计很独特。

2017-4b 号罐 360 度旋转视频二维码

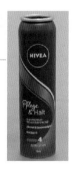

编号：2017-4c

英 文 介 绍

Can No. 4c: BDF Care & Hold

Marketed Can

Description: This is a series of cans in different formats. The center-piece shows a soft curl of hair. The brushed aluminum shines through the blue curl and gives the design a touch of pearle scence. The extremly fine gradation is blending into the blue background colour which contrasts the shiny centre-piece. This perfect gradation is achieved by the use of a new polymerisation technology for printing plates. The combination of the polymerization technology and laser cut printing plates makes this design so unique.

中 文 介 绍 ————————————————————————————————————

4c 号罐:

已上市罐

产品说明:

这是一系列不同形状的罐子。罐体中心图案展示了一头柔软的卷发。经过抛光的铝制表面在蓝色卷发的映衬下闪闪发光,为设计增添了一抹珍珠般的光泽。极其细腻的渐变色完美地融入蓝色背景中,与闪亮的中心部分形成对比。这种完美的渐变效果是通过使用一种新的印版聚合工艺技术实现的。聚合技术与激光雕刻印版技术的结合使这个设计很独特。

2017-4c 号罐 360 度旋转视频二维码

编号:2017-5a

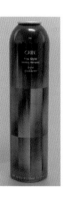

英 文 介 绍 ————————————————————————————————————

Can No. 5a:

Marketed Can

Description:

Oribe Free Styler Working Hairspray-(53 mm×205 mm)

All three sizes are manufactured using an oval shoulder profile, brushed surface and gold transparent base coating, dry offset printed graphics, gloss over varnish, 2Q pressure rating and gold PAM interior coating. Challenges for this family of items are many fold. Print quality, manufacturing of the cans and delivery are coordinated by two of the producers' manufacturing locations. Customer provides a mock-up sample created by their modelling agency for visual colour and graphic reproduction and used in their marketing materials. Graphics group has to interpolate the final artwork for the printed cans to match the artwork and visual appearance of the mock-up sample. As simple as the graphic might appear, this is a real challenge. The graphic elements are provided in CMYK which is the way the customer's mock-up sample is printed. The producer have to flatten the CMYK image into one spot colour "black" and each rectangular area in the artwork have to be modified to match the mock-up sample provided. Then he uses his dot gain curves designed for each press to manipulate the final dot sizes to reproduce the correct shade of colour. Not an easy task for sure. The application of the gold base coating is also a challenge since both manufacturing plants have to achieve the same colour value in their application. The producer uses a double hit plate technique to also make sure the density of the black ink at the top of each can is similar and also very dense. The use of digital plates and close attention to detail in graphics helps assure the project goes smoothly. Production staff does an excellent job in communication between two manufacturing sites, sharing information needed to make sure all three items matched. Overall, the customer is very happy with the final results and this new product launch has been a very big success.

中文介绍

5a 号罐:已上市罐

产品说明:

Oribe 自由造型头发定型喷雾剂,该罐尺寸规格为 53 mm×205 mm。

这个系列三种尺寸的产品均采用椭圆形肩部轮廓、拉丝表面和金色透明底涂层、干胶印图案、光油、2Q 压力等级以及金色 PAM 内涂层。这个系列产品面临诸多挑战。印刷质量、罐子制造和交付由两个生产商的生产基地进行协调。客户仅提供了由他们自己的样机制作的一个模型样本,用于色彩对比和图案再现,并用于营销。负责图案的团队必须为印刷罐插入最终的图案,使图案和视觉外观相匹配。尽管图案看起来很简单,但这是一个真正的挑战。图案元素以 CMYK 格式提供,这是客户提供样品的印刷方式。生产商必须将 CMYK 图像转换成一种专用"黑色",并且必须修改图像中的每个矩形区域以匹配所提供的模型样本。然后,他们使用网点增益曲线来控制最终的网点大小,以重现正确的色调。这无疑是一项艰巨的任务。金色底涂层的应用也是一个挑战,因为两个制造工厂必须在应用中达到相同的颜色值。生产商使用了双版套印技术,确保每个罐体顶部的黑色油墨的密度相似,且非常致密。数字印版的使用和对图形细节的密切关注有助于项目的顺利进行。生产人员在两个生产基地之间的沟通方面做得很好,共享了确保所有三个项目都匹配的所需信息。总体来说,客户对最终结果非常满意,新产品的推出取得了巨大成功。

2017-5a 号罐 360 度旋转视频二维码

编号:**2017-5b**

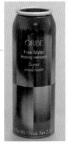

英文介绍

Can No. 5b:

Marketed Can

Description: Oribe Free Styler Working Hairspray (Travel Size: 38 mm×106 mm)

All three sizes are manufactured using an oval shoulder profile, brushed surface and gold transparent base coating, dry offset printed graphics, gloss over varnish, 2Q pressure rating and gold PAM interior coating. Challenges for this family of items are many fold. Print quality, manufacturing of the cans and delivery are coordinated by two of the producers' manufacturing locations. Customer provides a mock-up sample created by their modelling agency for visual colour and graphic reproduction and used in their marketing materials. Graphics group has to interpolate the final artwork for the printed cans to match the artwork and visual appearance of the mock-up sample. As simple as the graphic might appear, this is a real challenge. The graphic elements are provided in CMYK which is the way the customer's mock-up sample is printed. The producer have to flatten the CMYK image into one spot colour "black" and each rectangular area in the artwork have to be modified to match the mock-up sample provided. Then he uses his dot gain curves designed for each press to manipulate the final dot sizes to reproduce the correct shade of colour. Not an easy task for sure. The application of the gold base coating is also a challenge since both manufacturing plants have to achieve the same colour value in their application. The producer uses a double hit plate technique to also make sure the density of the black ink at the top of each can is similar and also very dense. The use of digital plates and close attention to detail in graphics helps assure the project goes smoothly. Production staff did an excellent job in communication between two manufacturing sites, sharing information needed to make sure all three items matched. Overall, the customer is very happy with the final results and this new product launch has been a very big success.

中文介绍

中文介绍:

5b 号罐:

已上市罐

产品说明:

　　Oribe 自由造型头发定型喷雾剂,该罐尺寸规格为 38 mm×106 mm(旅行装)。

　　这个系列三种尺寸的产品均采用椭圆形肩部轮廓、拉丝表面和金色透明底涂层、干胶印图案、光油、2Q 压力等级以及金色 PAM 内涂层。这个系列产品面临诸多挑战。印刷质量、罐子制造和交付由两个生产商的生产基地进行协调。客户仅提供了由他们自己的样机制作的一个模型样本,用于色彩对比和图案再现,并用于营销。负责图案的团队必须为印刷罐插入最终的图案,使图案和视觉外观相匹配。尽管图案看起来很简单,但这是一个真正的挑战。图案元素以 CMYK 格式提供,这是客户提供样品的印刷方式。生产商必须将 CMYK 图像转换成一种专用"黑色",并且必须修改图像中的每个矩形区域以匹配所提供的模型样本。然后,他使用网点增益曲线来控制最终的网点大小,以重现正确的色调。这无疑是一项艰巨的任务。金色底涂层的应用也是一个挑战,因为两个制造工厂必须在应用中达到相同的颜色值。生产商使用了双版套印技术,确保每个罐体顶部的黑色油墨的密度相似,且非常致密。数字印版的使用和对图形细节的密切关注有助于项目的顺利进行。生产人员在两个生产基地之间的沟通方面做得很好,共享了确保所有三个项目都匹配的所需信息。总体来说,客户对最终结果非常满意,新产品的推出取得了巨大成功。

2017-5b 号罐 360 度旋转视频二维码

编号:2017-5c

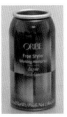

英文介绍

Can No. 5c:

Marketed Can

Description: Oribe Free Styler Working Hairspray(Purse Size: 38 mm×76 mm)

All three sizes are manufactured using an oval shoulder profile, brushed surface and gold transparent base coating, dry offset printed graphics, gloss over varnish, 2Q pressure rating and gold PAM interior coating. Challenges for this family of items are many fold. Print quality, manufacturing of the cans and delivery are coordinated by two of the producers' manufacturing locations. Customer provides a mock-up sample created by their modelling agency for visual colour and graphic reproduction and used in their marketing materials. Graphics group has to interpolate the final artwork for the printed cans to match the artwork and visual appearance of the mock-up sample. As simple as the graphic might appear, this is a real challenge. The graphic elements are provided in CMYK which is the way the customer's mock-up sample is printed. The producer have to flatten the CMYK image into one spot colour "black" and each rectangular area in the artwork have to be modified to match the mock-up sample provided. Then he uses his dot gain curves designed for each press to manipulate the final dot sizes to reproduce the correct shade of colour. Not an easy task for sure. The application of the gold base coating is also a challenge since both manufacturing plants have to achieve the same colour value in their application. The producer uses a double hit plate technique to also make sure the density of the black ink at the top of each can is similar and also very dense. The use of digital plates and close attention to detail in graphics helps assure the project goes smoothly. Production staff does an excellent job in communication between two manufacturing sites, sharing information needed to make sure all three items matched. Overall, the customer is very happy with the final results and this new product launch has been a very big success.

中文介绍

5c 号罐:

已上市罐

产品说明:

Oribe 自由造型头发定型喷雾剂,该罐尺寸规格为 38 mm×76 mm(钱包尺寸)。

这个系列三种尺寸的产品均采用椭圆形肩部轮廓、拉丝表面和金色透明底涂层、干胶印图案、光油、2Q 压力等级以及金色 PAM 内涂层。这个系列产品面临诸多挑战。印刷质量、罐子制造和交付由两个生产商的生产基地进行协调。客户仅提供了由他们自己的样机制作的一个模型样本,用于色彩对比和图案再现,并用于营销。负责图案的团队必须为印刷罐插入最终的图案,使图案和视觉外观相匹配。尽管图案看起来很简单,但这是一个真正的挑战。图案元素以 CMYK 格式提供,这是客户提供样品的印刷方式。生产商必须将 CMYK 图像转换成一种专用"黑色",并且必须修改图像中的每个矩形区域以匹配所提供的模型样本。然后,他使用网点增益曲线来控制最终的网点大小,以重现正确的色调。这无疑是一项艰巨的任务。金色底涂层的应用也是一个挑战,因为两个制造工厂必须在应用中达到相同的颜色值。生产商使用了双版套印技术,确保每个罐体顶部的黑色油墨的密度相似,且非常致密。数字印版的使用和对图形细节的密切关注有助于项目的顺利进行。生产人员在两个生产基地之间的沟通方面做得很好,共享了确保所有三个项目都匹配的所需信息。总体来说,客户对最终结果非常满意,新产品的推出取得了巨大成功。

2017-5c 号罐 360 度旋转视频二维码

编号:2017-6

英文介绍

Can No. 6: Anise Cosmetics, LLC Nail-Aid Aceton Spray Nail Polish Remover Keratin & Cocoa Butter

Marketed Can

Description: This can has 6 fl oz, 53 mm×175 mm, featuring comfort hold shoulder/body design, white base coating, dry offset printed graphics, gloss over varnish, 2Q pressure rating and gold epoxy phenolic interior coating. Challenge for this item is the prediction of distortion needed in the comfort hold or shaped area of the can. The customer wants a round graphic pattern reproduced and the text in that area needed to be undistorted on the final can. Fortunately, the producer is able to use his 3D modelling software to predict the distortion amount needed in the necked area of the can and accomplishes a much more rounded pattern by distorting the original graphic image provided. A 3D mock-up of the final can is produced with the customer's graphics wrapped around the final can shape. The customer loves the 3D proof and approves the final graphics so that the producer can proceed with print production of the job. When the image printed on the unformed can, it looks oval and it really puzzled litho operators until they see the final results on the formed can. The colour separation for the cocoa nuts and leaf image is done using a unique colour blending technique. The producer uses the customer's file prepared as a CMYK image and develops a separation using Pantone spot colours for added vibrancy on the printed can. Then the producer's proprietary dry dot screening technique is used to produce a separation that would print clean during the long press run. Once the plate ready file is prepared, dot gain curves are used to manipulate the final files used for digital plate making and the press to achieve the predicted result. Production staff does an outstanding job at matching the proofs shared with the customer for approval and maintained this quality throughout the run. There are also two other varieties of this product which followed similar artwork preparation and the customer is very happy with the outcome of all three items.

中文介绍

6 号罐:

已上市罐

产品说明:

该罐可装 6 盎司、53 mm×175 mm,具有舒适握持的肩部/罐身设计、白色底涂层、干胶印图案、高光油、2Q 压力等级以及金色环氧酚醛内涂层。这个项目的挑战是预测罐子的舒适握持或成形区所需的变形量。客户希望在最终罐体上重现一个"圆形"图案,并且该区域的文字不变形。幸运的是,生产商能够使用他的 3D 建模软件来预测罐颈区域所需的扭曲量,并通过扭曲原始图像来制作更圆润的图案,最终制作出罐体的 3D 模型,将客户的图案环绕在罐体形状上。

客户喜欢 3D 模型,并确认了最终的图案,这样生产商就可以继续进行印刷工作了。当在未成型的罐体上印刷图像时,它看起来是椭圆形的,这让胶印操作员非常困惑,直到他们看到成型罐体上的最终效果。可可豆和可可叶图像的分色使用了一种独特的色彩混合技术。生产商使用客户准备的文本作为 CMYK 格式文件,并使用潘通专色在印刷罐上进行分色,以增加印刷罐上的色彩饱和度。然后,生产商使用专有的干网点筛选技术用于制作分色版,以便在长时间印刷过程中保持清晰干净。一旦准备好印版文件,就使用网点增益曲线来处理用于数字制版和印刷的最终文件,以实现预期的结果。生产人员在匹配提供给客户审批的打样方面表现得非常出色,并在整个生产过程中保持其品质。该产品还有另外两个品种,采用了类似的图案,客户对这三个项目的结果都非常满意。

2017-6 号罐 360 度旋转视频二维码

编号:**2017-7**

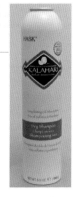

英文介绍

Can No. 7: Inspired Beauty Brands—Hask Kalahari Dry Shampoo

Marketed Can

Description: This can has 6. 5 oz 53 mm×220 mm, oval shoulder, white base coating, dry offset printed graphics, matte over varnish, 2P pressure rating, and gold epoxy phenolic interior coating. Challenge for this item is the pastel colour of the background of the can. This requires special attention during ink curing to maintain the colour throughout the production run. Also, pre-press proofing proves to be valuable since proofs help to predict the final visual reproduction of the artwork and the customer wants to make last minute changes to the soft screened graphics surrounding the centre logo on the front panel. Exact registration of the brown coloured small text on the back panel and front panel also are very difficult design requirements. Once the plate ready file is prepared the producer uses dot gain curves to manipulate the final files used for digital plate making and the press to achieve the predicted result. Production staff does an outstanding job at matching the proofs shared with the customer for approval and maintained this quality throughout the run. There are also four other varieties of this product which followed similar artwork preparation and the customer is very happy with the outcome of all five items.

中文介绍

7 号罐：

已上市罐

产品说明：

　　该罐重 6.5 盎司、53 mm×220 mm,椭圆形肩、白色底涂层、干胶印图案、哑光光油、2P 压力等级以及金色环氧酚醛内涂层。这个项目的挑战是罐体背景的柔和色彩。这需要特别注意油墨的固化过程,以便在整个生产过程中保持这种颜色。此外,印刷前打样被证明是有价值的,因为打样有助于预测图案的最终视觉效果,而且客户希望在最后一刻对罐体前面中心标志周围的图形进行更改。正面和背面棕色小文本的精准对齐也是非常困难的设计要求。一旦准备好印版文件,生产商使用网点增益曲线来处理用于数字制版和印刷的最终文件,以达到预期的结果。生产人员在匹配提供给客户审批的打样方面表现非常出色,并在整个生产过程中保持同样的品质。该系列还有其他四款产品,具有相似的图案设计,客户对这五个项目的结果都非常满意。

2017-7 号罐 360 度旋转视频二维码

编号：2017-8

英文介绍

Can No. 8: TAG Body Spray

Marketed Can

Description: MY Import USA LLC has recently relaunched a custom shaped aluminium aerosol can. The technical aspects of this container design incorporated aligned splined sections along with a recessed form area which is contoured to allow the "TAG" brand to be printed within the shape. This innovative design promotes exceptional shelf presence, provides product identity and aids in the elimination of product counterfeiting.

中 文 介 绍

8 号罐：

已上市罐

产品说明：

MY Import USA LLC 最近重新推出了一款定制形状的铝制喷雾罐。该容器的设计采用了对齐的锯齿状部分以及凹陷的成型区域，使 TAG 品牌的标志能够在该形状内印刷。这种创新的设计能够提升产品在货架上的展示效果，提高了产品的品牌标识功能，并有助于消除产品仿冒。

2017−8 号罐 360 度旋转视频二维码

编号：**2017−9**

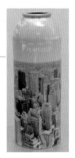

英 文 介 绍

Can No. 9: Printed Can Comparable to Digital Printing Prototypes Can

Description: With existing technical cabalities at the moment whether analogue or digital printing plates are produced with a resolution 2 540−4 000 ppi. With dry off-set printing technique inks will be used together at once and that results in general smearing of colours. Sample can used to send for the competition is printed only by using 4 colours CMYK(cyan-magenta-yellow and key black). All little details on the picture are reached nicely without smearing different inks. With this ideal result artwork and end result on the can itself matches perfectly.

More technical information:

For this can computer to plate cliches are printed with 5 080 ppi with other words with 157 line pi.

In order to hinder any smearing underneath of black colour is knocked-out so that CMY colours are printed on white base directly. This way black and other CMY do not come to a contact which creates smearings on printed cans.

Of course, very accurate registration of each printing plate is also required to obtain a clear picture in the end.

中 文 介 绍

9 号罐：

样品罐

产品说明：

目前，无论是模拟还是数字印刷版，其分辨率均为 2 540～4 000 ppi。采用凸版胶印技术，由于多种颜色的油墨同时使用,会导致颜色串色。用于比赛的样品罐仅使用 CMYK 四分色即青色、品红色、黄色和关键的黑色四种颜色进行印刷。图案上的所有小细节都达到了完美的效果,没有不同颜色油墨的混合扩散。这种理想的效果使图案和罐体的匹配非常完美。

更多技术信息:

为了防止串色导致的糊版,将黑色部分去掉,以便直接在白色底涂层上打印 CMY 颜色。这样,黑色和其他 CMY 就不会接触,也不会在印刷罐上产生扩散。当然,为了获得清晰的图像,每个印刷版的精确定位也是必不可少的。

2017-9 号罐 360 度旋转视频二维码

编号:2017-10

英文介绍

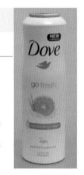

Can No. 10: Dove Go Fresh

Marketed Can

Description: Due to the ever increasing demand by customers for superior and more complex print designs, printing equipment has been developed over the past decade from the original standard 6 colour printing machine to the current 8 to 9 colour machines. These new developments however come at a significant cost to the can maker and in many developing markets this is not financially viable due to the low production volumes. This situation has left many customers at a competitive disadvantage as they have not being able to compete globally with the latest trends in print complexity and innovation. The producer has, however, introduced an innovative "twin ink duct" system on their original 6 colour polytype printing machines allowing them to develop and comfortably produce 7 or 8 colour designs on the current 6 inking units of the original polytype machine. This has given the customer the ability to standardise the quality of their product offering globally.

The "twin ink duct" system ensures that the production costs are contained and maximum benefit can be extracted from the current production equipment. This contains capital investment costs by extending the product life cycle of the current equipment.

This system differs from the traditional "split duct" system as it makes use of two smaller and completely separate ink ducts fitted to one printing deck. This eliminates the possibility of ink contamination in the ink duct with two different coloured inks in one unit. Further, the twin ink duct system also allows for complete control over the ink quantity and distribution in each duct. The innovation has additional benefits as it makes use of split ink roller sets to further assist in complete control over the two inks being run in printing deck. Split rollers prevent ink contamination on the rollers ensuring the colour and print quality is maintained during commercial production.

中文介绍

10 号罐：

已上市罐

产品说明：

　　由于客户对更高品质和复杂印刷设计的需求不断增加,在过去的十年里,印刷设备从最初的标准 6 色印刷机发展到现在的 8 到 9 色印刷机。然而,这些新发展给罐子制造商带来了巨大的成本压力,而且在许多新兴市场,由于产量低,入不敷出,经济上不可行。这种情况使许多客户在竞争处于不利地位,因为他们无法与全球最新的复杂和创新的印刷新趋势进行竞争。然而,生产商在原来的 6 色多型印刷机上引入了创新的双油墨管道系统,使他们能够在当前多型印刷机的 6 个油墨单元上开发并容易地生产 7 种或 8 种颜色的产品。这使客户有能力在全球范围内制定他们的产品质量标准。"双墨管道"系统确保生产成本可控,并从当前的生产设备中得到最大效益。这包含了通过延长现有设备的生命周期来控制资本的投资。

　　该系统不同于传统的"分体式管道"系统,因为它使用了安装在一个印刷平台上的两个更小的、完全独立的油墨管道。这消除了两种不同颜色的油墨在同一个油墨管道中互相污染的可能性。此外,双墨管道系统还能完全控制每个管道中油墨的数量及其分布。该创新还利用分体式油墨辊组,可以完全控制在印刷板上运行的两种油墨。分体式辊子可防止油墨之间的污染,有利于在商业生产过程中保持图案的色彩和印刷质量。

2017-10 号罐 360 度旋转视频二维码

编号：2017-12

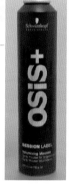

英文介绍

Can No. 12: OSiS+ Matte & Gloss

Marketed Can

Description: The OSiS+ Matte & Gloss aluminium aerosol can with flat shoulder is a testament to a package design created to reflect the desired user. The OSiS+ end user is a contemporary woman who seeks to achieve an understated signature style. The OSiS+ aerosol hairspray cans, in the black and brushed metal for mousse, are hardly overworked designs. Their crisp labels, which run vertically up the can, have an appealing clean aesthetic. By incorporating Matte & Gloss printing technology on the black OSiS+ Volumizing Mousse, the can has a modern, edgy feel. There is contrast between the glossy black (and glossy brushed silver logo) and the matte black background. The bold and sharp gloss black triangles are engaging and inviting the shopper to look and touch the can.

中文介绍

12 号罐：

已上市罐

产品说明：

OSiS+哑光亮面铝平肩气雾剂罐设计是包装设计的典范,旨在反映用户的需求。OSiS+的目标用户是追求低调独特风格的当代女性。OSiS+的黑色和磨砂金属材质的喷雾发胶罐几乎没有过度的设计。它们垂直地印刷在罐体上的向上延伸的清爽标签,有一种吸引人的简洁美感。在黑色 OSiS+丰盈定型摩丝罐上应用哑光亮面印刷技术,使罐体拥有现代、前卫的美感,亮面银色徽标和哑光黑色背景之间的对比鲜明,引人注目。大胆而锐利的哑光黑色三角形图案很吸引人,让消费者忍不住查看和触摸罐体。

2017-12 号罐 360 度旋转视频二维码

编号:2017-13

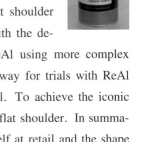

英文介绍

Can No. 13: L'oreal Men Expert Heat Protect

Marketed Can

Description: The new L'oreal Men Expert antiperspirant can employs innovative ReAl technology. This complex shape is executed on a 50 mm diameter flat shoulder can and run on 80-station necker. The 80-station machine is purchased with the development of ReAl in mind. This necking capability allows to drive ReAl using more complex shapes like the Men Expert 200 mL and 250 mL cans. It also paves the way for trials with ReAl Gen2 with even more recycled content and greater lightweighting potential. To achieve the iconic shape of this can body there is diameter reduction and re-expansion with a flat shoulder. In summation, the bold orange on the aluminium aerosol can leaps out from the shelf at retail and the shape provides aesthetic and ergonomic comfort for the consumer.

中文介绍

13 号罐：

已上市罐

产品说明：

全新的欧莱雅男士专用防汗剂喷雾罐采用了创新的 ReAl 专利技术。这个罐复杂的形状是在一个直径 50 mm 的叙肩罐、80 工位的缩颈机上完成的。购买这台 80 工位的机器时专门为开发 ReAl 技术而购买的。这种缩颈功能允许驱动 ReAl 形成更复杂的形状，如男士专用 200 mL 和 250 mL 的气雾罐。它还为 ReAl Gen2 的试验铺平了道路，ReAl Gen2 具有更多的可回收成分和更大的轻量化潜力。为了达到这个罐体的经典形状，罐身的成型经历了直径的缩小和肩型的再扩张。总而言之，具有醒目橙色的铝制气雾罐在零售货架上跃然而出，其形状为消费者提供了美学和人体工程学的舒适感。

2017-13 号罐 360 度旋转视频二维码

编号：2017-14

英 文 介 绍

Can No. 14: 360°

Prototypes Can

Description: Symmetrical and asymmetrical shaping is available up to the full circumference of the can. The artwork can be oriented to the relief area which complements the shaping. This can is visually engaging from all angles while providing additional grip for usability.

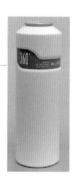

中 文 介 绍

14 号罐：

样品罐

产品说明：

可提供对称和非对称的罐身造型，直至罐身的整个圆周。图案可定向至凸起区域，以增强罐身的造型效果。这种罐子从各个角度看都非常吸引人，同时提供了更好的握持性。

2017-14 号罐 360 度旋转视频二维码

编号：2017-15

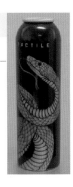

英文介绍

Can No. 15: Tactile

Prototypes Can

Description: Tactile or raised ink offers textured grip for unique consumer interaction with the package. The tactile pattern can be applied on 360 degrees of the can and can be designed and applied in a particular pattern, resembling snakeskin, honeycomb or the skin of an orange etc.

中文介绍

15 号罐：

样品罐

产品说明：

触觉或凸起的油墨为消费者提供了与包装的独特互动。触感图案可以应用在罐体的 360 度上，并且可以设计和应用于像蛇皮、蜂窝或橙子皮等类似的特定图案。

2017-15 号罐 360 度旋转视频二维码

编号：2017-16

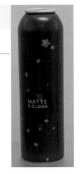

英文介绍

Can No. 16: Matte & Gloss

Prototypes Can

Description: Matte & Gloss technology combines matte and gloss finishes on the same can, creating a striking visual presentation. The distinct contrast between the reflective gloss and soft, subdued matte finish is ideal for darker colours. The producers new matte and gloss process offers improved ink lay, offering even more contrast between the matte and gloss.

中文介绍

16 号罐：

样品罐

产品说明：

哑光与亮光技术将哑光和亮光两种印刷结合在同一个罐子上，创造出引人惊叹的视觉效果。亮光的反射光泽与柔和低调的哑光之间的鲜明对比非常理想。制造商用新型哑光与亮光工艺为油墨提供了更好的附着力,使哑光与亮光之间的对比更加鲜明。

2017-16 号罐 360 度旋转视频二维码

编号:2017-17

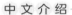

英文介绍

Can No. 17: Double Wall Can

Prototypes Can

Description: The can is double-walled and can be decorated both outside and inside. With this push-on-cap can we want to show how well we can handle the material aluminium and the production process "impact extrusion", also with regard to our ever-growing aerosol can production. The double wall can is a promotion article on our own account and can be produced in all diameters.

中文介绍

17 号罐:

样品罐

产品说明:

  该罐为双层夹壁式结构,内外均可装饰。通过这款采用压入式推盖罐展示我们在生产过程中处理铝材和冲击挤压工艺的卓越能力。双层夹壁式罐是我们自有的促销产品,可以制成各种直径的罐体。

2017-17 号罐 360 度旋转视频二维码

编号:2017-18

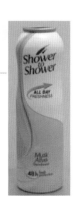

英文介绍

Can No. 18: Shower to Shower Deodorant

Marketed Can

Description: Shaping is one of the major brand building packaging solutions available to marketers seeking to develop an imaginatively designed and functional package. It allows marketers the ability to create a competitive advantage through product differentiation. The producer developed a unique shape specifically for Amka products to represent their female range of deodorants. The shower deodorant can makes use of soft flowing curves to give a very feminine feel that ergonomically fits well in the user's hand. To further enhance the visual impact of this aerosol, the decoration artwork has been developed to fit perfectly with an accentuate and complement the flowing shape of the can. As a finishing touch, a semi matte over varnish is applied to create a luxurious touch for the end consumer.

This shaped can takes material savings into consideration by making use of a very stable shoulder profile resistant to collapsing under shaping and filling top loads. Further, it lends itself to material reduction/light weighting ensuring effective use and reduction of raw material resources. The tooling and development cost is also kept to a minimum by maximising on the capabilities of the existing tooling.

The design parameters of the shaping tools are carefully considered to ensure that they do not exceed the standard necking machine stroke length capability. This allows production to proceed at normal/full speed with no penalty in production throughput. Standard necking machines can be used to produce this can, eliminating the need for high capital investment in new equipment as well as enabling flexibility in the manufacturing process as this shaped can can be produced on several standard production lines. Inherent production defects related to shaped cans are eliminated/kept to a minimum due to the flowing shape of the tooling ensuring low spoilage and minimizing production stoppages from the necking process. This allows the lowest possible production costs for such a shaped product.

中文介绍

18 号罐：

已上市罐

产品说明：

造型是营销人员寻求开发具有创意设计和功能包装的主要品牌建设解决方案之一。它使营销人员能够通过产品差异化创造竞争优势。制造商为 Amka 产品开发了独特的造型,以代表其女性香体剂系列。沐浴香体剂罐采用柔和流畅的曲线,给人一种非常女性化的感觉,符合人体工程学,适合用户抓握。为了进一步增强这种喷雾剂的视觉冲击力,罐体上的装饰图案被精心设计,完美地配合罐体流线的形状,相辅相成。作为最后的点缀,应用了一种半哑光油,为最终消费者创造出奢华的感觉。

这种罐体通过使用非常稳定的肩部轮廓来节省材料,防止在成型和顶部受压下坍塌变形。此外,它有助于减少材料/减轻重量,确保有效使用和减少原材料资源。通过充分利用现有模具的功能,最大限度地降低了新模具的开发成本。制造商需要认真考虑成型工具的设计参数,以确保它们不超过标准缩颈机的运行长度。这使得生产以正常速度/全速进行,而不会影响产量。标准缩颈机可用于生产这种罐体,省略了对新设备的高成本投资,并使生产线具有灵活性。因为这种成型罐头可以在多个标准生产线上生产。由于工具的流动形状确保了低废品率和最小化缩颈过程的生产停顿,从而消除了与成型罐头相关的固有生产缺陷,并使生产成本降至最低。

2017-18 号罐 360 度旋转视频二维码

九、2016年国际铝气雾罐竞赛参赛罐

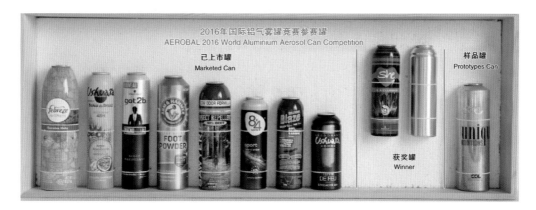

罐编号从左至右分别是:9,1,11,6,7,3,5,2,10,4,8

编号:2016-1

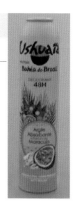

英文介绍

Can No. 1: Ushuaia Femme

Marketed

Description: A bright colourful aerosol can that emits the feeling of beach and sunshine. The printing technique used in this design successfully portrays the artistic realism of the passion fruit. The design is remarkably detailed. For example, the palm leaf is proof of this master printing. Every small dot is precisely at its place and has a perfect contour. The clear contour is achieved by a new laser prepress process. The printing blocks are produced extremely accurate and thus making extremely fine and perfect designs possible without loss of quality.

中文介绍

1 号罐:

已上市罐

产品说明:

　　这是一款色彩鲜艳的气雾剂罐,散发出沙滩和阳光的感觉。这个设计中使用的印刷技术成功描绘了百香果的艺术写实效果。这个设计非常精美绝伦,如棕榈叶就是这种精湛印刷技术的证明。每一个小点都精确地位于其应有的位置,具有完美的轮廓。清晰的轮廓是通过一种新的激光印刷工艺实现的。印版制作得非常精确,因此可以实现无损质量的精细和完美的设计。

2016-1 号罐 360 度旋转视频二维码

编号：**2016-2**

英文介绍

Can No. 2: Ushuaia Homme

Marketed Can

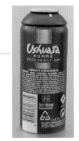

Description: A new range of deodorants for men with a metallic brown base colour and eye-catching centre pieces. The combination of translucent and opaque inks proves to be a real challenge. The translucent centre piece has to be aligned with the opaque ink in such a way that both inks don't mix, yet there is no gap visible in the design. A translucent ink on top of an opaque ink will result in an unwanted discoloration. The gradient from opaque to translucent is done to perfection, there is no discolouration visible.

The centre piece of the Ushuaia can is printed by a special printing technique, which is unique, and also taking the ink rheology into account. This means the consistency of the ink is taken into account during the print process. A translucent ink is more liquid than the opaque ink. And the art is to anticipate the fluidity of the translucent and opaque ink to a defined point according to the design. This centre piece shows the perfect combination of repro artwork, computer to plate, ink preparation and the print process itself. The composition of the artwork has to be done in such a way that inks bond with the can body but also with other layers of ink. In order to achieve the fine gradients, translucency in some cans the negative printing of the centre piece the inks has to be applied in a very special "layered" printing technique.

中文介绍

2 号罐：

已上市罐

产品说明：

这是一款为男士设计的新型香体剂系列，罐身以金属棕色为底色，配有引人注目的中心装饰。透明和不透明油墨的组合是一个真正的挑战。透明的中央图案必须与不透明的油墨完美对齐，以便两种墨水不会混合，且在设计中没有明显的缝隙。在不透明的油墨上加半透明的油墨会出现无法预料的色差。从不透明到半透明的渐变处理得恰到好处，没有任何可见的色差。

Ushuaia 罐体的中心图案采用了一种特殊的印刷技术，这种印刷技术不仅独特，也考虑了油墨的流变性。这意味着在印刷过程中要考虑油墨的黏稠度。透明油墨比不透明油墨更液态。其技巧在于根据设计要求将半透明和不透明油墨的流动性调整到一个特定点。这个中心图案展示了从电脑制版、油墨准备到印刷过程本身的完美结合。图案中的油墨不仅要与罐身相结合,也要与其他层的油墨相结合。为了达到精细的渐变的半透明效果,在一些罐体中,中心图案的负片印刷必须采用非常特殊的"分层"印刷技术。

2016-2 号罐 360 度旋转视频二维码

编号:2016-3

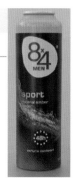

英 文 介 绍

Can No. 3: 8×4 Men Sport

Marketed Can

Description: It is a masculine can that shows a remarkable print design. The printing technique utilized in this design shows extraordinary craftsmanship. The dark background, containing a high concentration of pigments, gives a remarkable contrast to the turquoise-coloured gush of water that acts as centrepiece. The matt background enhances the metallic centrepiece. To achieve this effect the manufacturer has to build up the colours in a very specific way and order. Only this printing technique results in this fabulous look. Very few manufacturers can do this to this extent. The fine gradient at the base of the can and the silver print of letters achieved with negative print technique complements the can very well.

中 文 介 绍

3 号罐:

已上市罐

产品说明:

这是一款设计精美的男士运动饮料罐。该设计中使用的印刷技术展示了非凡的工艺水平。深色背景中含有高浓度颜料,与图案中心作为点缀的翠绿色的水流形成了鲜明的对比。哑光背景增强了金属的质感。为了达到这种效果,制造商必须以一种非常特殊的方式和顺序来构建颜色。只有这种印刷技术才能呈现这种美妙的外观。几乎没有制造商能做到这种效果,罐体底部的精细渐变和负片印刷技术的银色字母相得益彰,使罐体看起来很完美。

2016-3 号罐 360 度旋转视频二维码

编号:2016-4

Can No. 4: Purity

Prototypes Can

Description:

A new way of manufacturing aerosol can.

The first aerosol cans without any inner and outer coating out of aluminium. The patent pending Purity can production process turns the existing standard up-side down.

Extrusion, cutting/trimming and brushing, necking, washing.

The specification of the can has not been altered and yet the can has improved qualities. Side effects of those changes are: same spec, higher burst pressure, less energy, less CO_2, less machine investment, shorter production cycle.

4 号罐:

样品罐

产品说明:

一种制造气雾罐的新方法。

首款没有任何内外涂层的铝制气雾罐。正在申请专利的 Purity 罐,其生产工艺颠覆了现有的标准。

冲压、切割/修边和刷涂、缩颈、清洗。

罐的规格没有改变,但罐子的质量却得到了改善。这些变化还带来了附带的效果:相同的规格下具更高的爆破压力、更少的能源消耗、更少的二氧化碳排放、更少的机械投资以及更短的生产周期。

2016-4 号罐 360 度旋转视频二维码

编号:2016-5

Can No. 5: Blaze Ant, Roach & Earwig Killer

Marketed Can

Description: This can has 100 g, 45 mm×150 mm, round shoulder, 9-colour graphics printed over a white base coating.

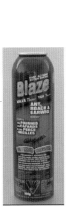

中 文 介 绍

5 号罐:

已上市罐

产品说明:

　　该罐可装 100 g,45 mm×150 mm,圆形肩部,在白色底涂层上印有 9 色图案。

2016-5 号罐 360 度旋转视频二维码

编号:**2016-6**

英 文 介 绍

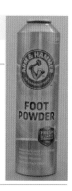

Can No. 6: Arm & Hammer Foot Powder

Marketed Can

Description: Arm & Hammer foot powder spray with fresh guard, 7.5 oz, 53 mm× 185 mm, flat deg shoulder, 9-colour graphics with silver glitter base coating.

中 文 介 绍

6 号罐:

已上市罐

产品说明:

　　手臂足部爽身喷雾,重 7.5 盎司、53 mm×185 mm,斜肩,在银光闪闪的底涂层上印有 9 色图案。

2016-6 号罐 360 度旋转视频二维码

编号:**2016-7**

英 文 介 绍

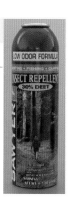

Can No. 7: Sawyer Insect Repellent

Marketed Can

Description: This can has 53 mm×175 mm, rounded shoulder, 9-colour graphics printed over a white base coating.

中 文 介 绍

7 号罐：

已上市罐

产品说明：

该罐 53 mm×175 mm，圆形肩部，在白色底涂层上印有 9 色图案。

2016-7 号罐 360 度旋转视频二维码

编号：2016-8

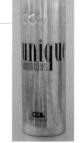

英 文 介 绍

Can No. 8: Unique

Prototypes Can

Description: It's a 53 mm×175 mm conical shoulder aerosol can. The producer offers the "de-bossed" design as an innovative option to "dial-in" a specific brand name or logo. The process allows brands to "highlight" a unique feature on the can which provides a focal point for greater consumer awareness. Spot de-bossing along with graphically orientated "direct" printing creates specific visual contact and intrigue.

中 文 介 绍

8 号罐：

样品罐

产品说明：

这是一款 53 mm×175 mm 和斜肩的气雾剂罐，生产商采用创新的"凹凸式浮雕"设计，可将一个特定的品牌名称或标志"嵌入"其中。这一制作方法使品牌能够在罐体上"突出"其独特的特征，从而成为吸引消费者注意的焦点。凹凸式浮雕以及专有图案的"直接"印刷，创造出特定的视觉接触和吸引力。

2016-8 号罐 360 度旋转视频二维码

编号：2016-9

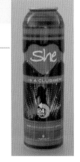

英文介绍

Can No. 9: Febreze Air Effects Hawaiian Aloha

Marketed Can

Description:

It's a 59 mm×201 mm trimline shoulder aerosol can.

The producer's computer to plate process has improved colour application developing crisp floral definition for multi-colour graphics. This aluminium container includes bright, eye catching, full coverage graphics which establishes distinction on retail shelves.

中文介绍

9 号罐：

已上市罐

产品说明：

这是一款 59 mm×201 mm 的带有线条修长肩型的气雾剂罐。

生产商运用电脑制版技术改进了色彩的应用,从而实现了清晰的花卉图案,适用于多色图形。这种铝制容器配有明亮醒目的全覆盖图案,使其在零售货架上脱颖而出。

2016-9 号罐 360 度旋转视频二维码

编号：2016-10

英文介绍

Can No. 10: She is a Clubber

Marketed Can

Description: Based on a request from the valued customer, Hunca Cosmetics in Turkey, the producer develops a brand new can design for their existing brand "she", which is very reputable in Turkey as well as Middle East. Due to the well-known brand, they have been encountering many counterfeits in the Middle East, as well as North Africa. So the producer has proposed them utilizing a printing oriented shaping technique. By this way, the producer manages to create a unique heart shape in front of the can, which enables them to allocate and highlight the brand "she" in the middle. On the back side of the can, the "she" brand is again emphasized by the asymmetrical rotation of the shaped area, which is provided by an orientation system. This unique and revolutionary design will protect the customers' products, avoiding counterfeits, which will surely boost their sales in the Middle East.

中文介绍

10 号罐:

已上市罐

产品说明:

  根据土耳其知名化妆品品牌 Hunca Cosmetics 的要求,生产商为其现有品牌"she"设计了一款全新的气雾剂罐造型,该品牌在土耳其和中东地区都享有盛誉。但由于其知名度高,在中东和北非地区也出现了许多假冒产品。因此,生产商建议他们采用一种以印刷为主的成型技术。生产商成功地在罐子正面创造了一个独特的心形图案,使他们能够在中间突出和强调"她"品牌。在罐体背面,"she"的品牌再次通过一个由定向系统提供的非对称旋转来实现。这种独特和革命性的设计将有效保护消费者的产品,避免假冒产品,也将大幅提升它们在中东地区的销量。

2016-10 号罐 360 度旋转视频二维码

编号:2016-11

英文介绍

Can No. 11: Henkel Schwarzkopf got2b

Marketed Can

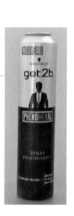

Description: The Henkel Schwarzkopf got2b extruded aluminium can's graphics are both simple and elegant, with distinct contrast between the reflective gloss and soft, subdued matte finishes.

  In the typical can decoration process the usual coater-rolling application of over-varnishes does not allow for separate areas of matte and gloss finish registered to the print. To a-chieve the final got2b MANN-O-MANN hairspray can Henkel Schwarzkopf works closely with the producer, who used specialized inks and coatings to achieve a matte or a gloss overvarnish finish in the different printed areas of the can.

  The new matte and gloss application can be run on standard printing and coating equipment using modified process parameters. This allows brand owners to accentuate different areas of the can for marketing purposes. Got2b accomplished this by highlighting the tuxedo depicted in the can decoration with a gloss varnish that pops against the predominantly matte can. This can's eye-catching graphics and distinctive presence stand out on the shelf and set this product apart from the competition.

中 文 介 绍

11 号罐:

已上市罐

产品说明:

汉高施华蔻 got2b 牌挤压铝罐的图案设计既简洁又优雅,具有明显的光泽与柔和哑光对比效果。

在传统的罐体印刷过程中,常规的涂布和滚涂覆膜工艺很难将哑光和亮光区域分享。为了达到最终的 got2b MANN-O-MANN 发胶罐的效果,汉高施华蔻与生产商密切合作,他们使用专用的油墨和涂层,在罐的不同印刷区域实现哑光或亮光的覆膜效果。

这种新的哑光和亮光的应用可以在标准印刷和涂层设备上通过修改工艺参数来实现。这使得品牌所有者可以突出罐体的不同区域,以达到营销目的。Got2b 在罐体正面设计了晚礼服图案,使其在以哑光为主的罐体上格外突出。这款罐体引人注目的图案和独特的外观在货架上很显眼,使该产品与竞争对手区分。

2016-11 号罐 360 度旋转视频二维码

十、2015 年国际铝气雾罐竞赛参赛罐

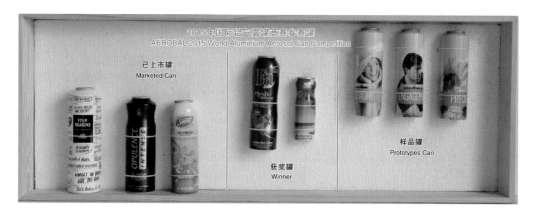

罐编号从左至右分别是:1,4,3,5,6,2,2-1,2-2

编号:**2015-1**

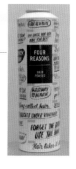

英文介绍

Can No. 1: Four Reasons

Marketed Can

Description: This can displays an unusual design. The brand "Four Reasons" shows 35 different "Reasons"—all numbered—about hair. A lot of the "Reasons" are altered song titles which makes this can really interesting to explore. The various typography is printed in a special black polyester ink on a white opaque background so the design resembles a newspaper. What looks so easy is proof of the special know-how to work with polyester ink, only this manufacuter has. In general alkyd colours are used for printing aerosol cans as they are less complecated to work with. To achieve sophisticated print designs with polyester ink the whole process has to be aligned from the printing cloth to the printing device and last but not least the training and expert know-how of the printing staff in order to achieve perfect decorations. The fresh green highlights and cap complement the overall look of this can.

中文介绍

1 号罐:

已上市罐

产品说明:

　　这款罐体展示了独特的设计。品牌"Four Reasons"展示了与头发有关的 35 个不同的"理由"全部编号。其中有些"理由"是经过改编的歌曲标题,这使得这款罐体特别有趣易引人探

究。各种字体采用特殊的黑色聚酯油墨印刷在白色不透明的背景上,使设计看起来像一张报纸。看似简单的设计,实际上展示了聚酯油墨所需的特殊专业知识,只有这家制造商拥有这种技术。通常由于醇酸颜料易于使用而用于印刷气雾罐。然而,用聚酯油墨实现复杂的印刷设计,需要从印刷涂布到印刷设备的整个过程进行协调以及对印刷人员专业技能的培训,以实现完美的装饰效果。鲜绿色的点缀与盖子使罐子的整体外观更加完美。

2015-1 号罐 360 度旋转视频二维码

编号:2015-2

英文介绍

Can No. 2: Eyeris

Prototypes Can

Description: Ball's proprietary Eyeris technique offers printing that will captivate customers, elevate their brand, and outshine their competition. Ball's unique approach to artwork separations, coupled with innovative plate-engraving techniques, 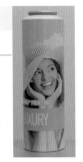 yields the most impressive graphics imaginable. This proprietary technique began in our beverage division and is now commercially available on aluminium aerosol cans. Eyeris produces near-digital quality printing without the need for the customer to invest in additional tooling or equipment. Laser engraving techniques are used to sculpt a variety of elevations into the plates allowing us to produce a variety of dot sizes on the same can. The result is an unprecedented level of detail easily overcoming challenging colours and textures for things like hair and shadows. Eyeris has been perfected for all can sizes and can utilize upwards of 8-color printing. The Eyeris cans submitted are designed and produced in Ball's plant in San Luis Potosi, Mexico.

中文介绍

2 号罐:

样品罐

产品说明:

　　Ball 公司独有的"Eyeris"技术可提供令人着迷的印刷效果,提升品牌形象并超越竞争对手。Ball 独特的图案分色方法,结合创新的雕版技术,创造出令人印象深刻的图案。这项专有技术始于我们的饮料部门,现已经在铝气雾罐上实现商业化应用。"Eyeris"技术能实现接近数字印刷的质量,而无需客户投资额外的工具或设备。激光雕刻技术用于在版面上雕刻各种深浅的纹理,使我们能够在同一罐体上制作一系列不同尺寸的点。其结果展现了一个无与伦比的细节,轻松克服了诸如头发和阴影等具有挑战性的颜色和纹理。Eyeris 技术适合各种尺寸的罐体,并支持多达 8 色的印刷。以上所述的 Eyeris 罐是在 Ball 公司位于墨西哥圣路易斯波托西的工厂设计和制造的。

2015-2 号罐 360 度旋转视频二维码

编号:2015-2-1

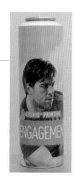

英文介绍

Can No. 2-1: Eyeris

Prototypes Can

Description: Ball's proprietary Eyeris technique offers printing that will captivate customers, elevate their brand, and outshine their competition. Ball's unique approach to artwork separations, coupled with innovative plate-engraving techniques, yields the most impressive graphics imaginable. This proprietary technique began in our beverage division and is now commercially available on aluminium aerosol cans. Eyeris produces near-digital quality printing without the need for the customer to invest in additional tooling or equipment. Laser engraving techniques are used to sculpt a variety of elevations into the plates allowing us to produce a variety of dot sizes on the same can. The result is an unprecedented level of detail easily overcoming challenging colours and textures for things like hair and shadows. Eyeris has been perfected for all can sizes and can utilize upwards of 8-color printing. The Eyeris cans submitted are designed and produced in Ball's plant in San Luis Potosi, Mexico.

中文介绍

2-1 号罐:

样品罐

产品说明:

　　Ball 公司独有的"Eyeris"技术可提供令人着迷的印刷效果,提升品牌形象并超越竞争对手。Ball 独特的图案分色方法,结合创新的雕版技术,创造出令人印象深刻的图案。这项专有技术始于我们的饮料部门,现已经在铝气雾罐上实现商业化应用。"Eyeris"技术能实现接近数字印刷的质量,而无需客户投资额外的工具或设备。激光雕刻技术用于在版面上雕刻各种深浅的纹理,使我们能够在同一罐体上制作一系列不同尺寸的点。其结果展现了一个无与伦比的细节,轻松克服了诸如头发和阴影等具有挑战性的颜色和纹理。Eyeris 技术适合各种尺寸的罐体,并支持多达 8 色的印刷。以上所述的 Eyeris 罐是在 Ball 公司位于墨西哥圣路易斯波托西的工厂设计和制造的。

2015-2-1号罐360度旋转视频二维码

编号:2015-2-2

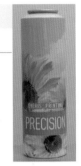

英文介绍

Can No. 2-2: Eyeris

Prototypes Can

Description: Ball's proprietary Eyeris technique offers printing that will captivate customers, elevate their brand, and outshine their competition. Ball's unique approach to artwork separations, coupled with innovative plate-engraving techniques, yields the most impressive graphics imaginable. This proprietary technique began in our beverage division and is now commercially available on aluminium aerosol cans. Eyeris produces near-digital quality printing without the need for the customer to invest in additional tooling or equipment. Laser engraving techniques are used to sculpt a variety of elevations into the plates allowing us to produce a variety of dot sizes on the same can. The result is an unprecedented level of detail easily overcoming challenging colours and textures for things like hair and shadows. Eyeris has been perfected for all can sizes and can utilize upwards of 8-color printing. The Eyeris cans submitted are designed and produced in Ball's plant in San Luis Potosi, Mexico.

中文介绍

2-2号罐:

样品罐

产品说明:

Ball 公司独有的"Eyeris"技术可提供令人着迷的印刷效果,提升品牌形象并超越竞争对手。Ball 独特的图案分色方法,结合创新的雕版技术,创造出令人印象深刻的图案。这项专有技术始于我们的饮料部门,现已经在铝气雾罐上实现商业化应用。"Eyeris"技术能实现接近数字印刷的质量,而无需客户投资额外的工具或设备。激光雕刻技术用于在版面上雕刻各种深浅的纹理,使我们能够在同一罐体上制作一系列不同尺寸的点。其结果展现了一个无与伦比的细节,轻松克服了诸如头发和阴影等具有挑战性的颜色和纹理。Eyeris 技术适合各种尺寸的罐体,并支持多达 8 色的印刷。以上所述的 Eyeris 罐是在 Ball 公司位于墨西哥圣路易斯波托西的工厂设计和制造的。

2015-2-2 号罐 360 度旋转视频二维码

编号: 2015-3

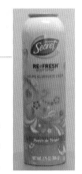

英 文 介 绍

Can No. 3: Secret Pasión de Tango

Marketed Can

Description: The "Secret Pasión de Tango" design requires a colour transition from blue to green to the white background colour. The producer is able to attain the proper appearance on the can using split ink wells along with careful ink flow control. The general crisp appearance of the artwork on the can is achieved using plates from a CTP process. With high intensity UV light, the producer is able to achieve a sharper edge that allows for smaller dots.

中 文 介 绍

3 号罐:

已上市罐

产品说明:

　　"Secret Pasión de Tango" 型的设计要求从蓝色到绿色再到白色背景色的渐变效果。生产商利用分体式油墨盒,并结合对油墨流量的精准控制,成功地实现了这一预期的外观效果。通过 CTP 工艺的制版,啤酒罐上的艺术图案可以实现清晰的整体效果。通过高强度的 UV 光,生产商可以实现更清晰的图案边缘,从而允许在印刷中使用更小的网点。

2015-3 号罐 360 度旋转视频二维码

编号: 2015-4

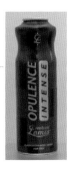

英 文 介 绍

Can No. 4: Création Lamis Opulence Intense

Marketed Can

Description: The producer offers a new printing technology, Matte & Gloss, which combines matte and gloss finishes on the same can. This creates a unique contrasting effect because the gloss reflects light while the matte absorbs it. This effect can grab and hold the consumer's attention.

In addition, this new printing process allows the client to design their cans in such a way that engages the consumer's senses of sight and touch. This new technique results in strong on-shelf differentiation from competitors and an improved consumer experience.

The Création Lamis demonstrates the capabilities of this technique through its checkered Matte & Gloss finish. The can is also designed to feature an ergonomic shape that complements the lithography technique, while providing an additional feature for the customer.

中文介绍

4 号罐:

已上市罐

产品说明:

生产商推出了一种新的印刷技术,能够在同一罐体上同时呈现哑光和亮光的效果。这创造了一种独特的对比效果,因为亮光反射光线,而哑光吸收光线。这种效果有效地吸引并抓住了消费者的注意力。

此外,这种创新的印刷工艺使生产商在设计罐体时能够兼顾消费者的视觉和触觉。这种新技术使产品在货架上与竞争对手形成了显著的差异,并且提高了消费者体验。

Création Lamis 通过其方格哑光和亮光的饰面展示了这项技术。此外,该罐的设计符合人体工程学,与平版印刷技术相辅相成,为消费者提供了另一个特色体验。

2015-4 号罐 360 度旋转视频二维码

编号:2015-5

英文介绍

Can No. 5: Fa Mystic Moments

Marketed Can

Description: The can producer and Henkel Beauty Care continue to pioneer sustainable aluminium aerosol packaging. With the release of the Fa ReAl can, the producer has succeeded in producing an ultra-lightweight (20 grams) aluminium aerosol can that has 25% recycled aluminium content. This metal alloy is stronger and lighter without affecting the package integrity. For a 150 mL and 200 mL sized can, Henkel's Fa is now the lightest commercially available can in the market. The producer estimates this lighter weight ReAl technology will result in a product carbon footprint reduction of 12%. Additionally, despite the increased alloy strength, the producer successfully developed a container with a deep shape to produce a can with a distinctive shelf presence. Everyone wins with ReAl—the customer, the consumer and the environment.

中文介绍

5 号罐：

已上市罐

产品说明：

　　罐体生产商和汉高美容护理公司一直处于可持续铝气雾罐包装的领先地位，随着 Fa 的 ReAl 罐的推出，生产商成功生产出一种超轻（20 g）铝气雾罐，其中含有 25% 的回收铝。这种先进的金属合金既坚固又轻便，且不会影响包装的完整性。在尺寸选择方面，对于容量为 150 mL 和 200 mL 的罐体，汉高的 Fa 系列现已成为市场上最轻的商用罐，这种更轻的 ReAl 技术的应用使商用罐的碳足迹减少 12%。此外，尽管它提高了合金强度，生产商还是成功开发了一种深型容器，以赋予罐体独特的货架展示效果。使用 ReAl 技术对客户、消费者和环境的每方都有益的。

2015-5 号罐 360 度旋转视频二维码

编号：**2015-6**

英文介绍

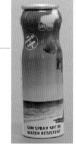

Can No. 6: Evolution Mini Shape Nussbaum Sun Spray (50 mL)

Prototypes Can

Description: Evolution mini shape printed with Nussbaum sun spray 50 mL (Promotion Can). The portfolio of the Evolution range has been extended by the promo size of the evolution mini can and with its 50 mL content the aluminium can offers the perfect travel size format. The ergonomically shaped waist profile provides an attractive packaging solution for personal care, pharmaceutical, technical or food products. The vibrancy of the photorealistic image has been produced with laser engraved printing plates. The Evolution range includes different diameters to accommodate volumes from 50 mL up to 250 mL. The Evolution mini can with 35 mm offers the ideal specification to fill 75 mL, a volume which is most suitable for using compressed can technology.

中文介绍

6 号罐：

样品罐

产品说明：

  该罐是 Evolution 系列的迷你型罐，印有 Nussbaum 太阳喷雾（50 mL）促销罐。Evolution 系列迷你罐扩大了系列产品的投资组合，引入了一个促销规格。这种铝罐具有 50 mL 的容量，非常适合旅行。其符合人体工程学的腰部轮廓为个人护理、制药、技术或食品产业提供了一个个有吸引力的包装解决方案。色彩鲜艳的逼真图像是通过激光雕刻印版来实现的。Evolution 系列包括各种直径规格，可容纳从 50 mL 到 250 mL 的容量。专门设计的直径为 35 mm 的 E-volution 迷你罐为 75 mL 提供了一个理想的容量规格，非常适合使用气雾罐技术。

2015-6 号罐 360 度旋转视频二维码

十一、2014 年国际铝气雾罐竞赛参赛罐

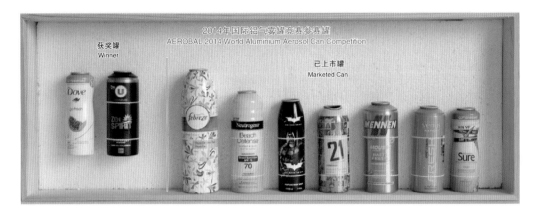

罐编号从左至右分别是:3,9,2,4,5,6,7,8,1

编号:2014-1

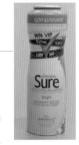

英 文 介 绍

Can No. 1: Sure Bright—Compressed Can

Marketed Can

Description: The can has a white base coat which shines through the design. The design consists of contrary raster patterns. One raster pattern starts at the base from dark pink to light pink and ends just above the headline Woman Sure. At approximately this height the direction of the raster pattern changes from an upward to a sideway direction. Displaying darker pink near the bands and a light pink towards the writing/back of the can. The leaves are printed in every shade of pink from a very small size to a bigger size. The innovation of the can lies also in its content—125 mL will last as long as a 250 mL deo can. This means less material, less weight and less transport cost—but still an elegant can.

中 文 介 绍

1 号罐:

已上市罐

产品说明:

　　该罐具有白色底涂层,使设计图案更加醒目。该设计采用了对比强烈的网格图案。其中一个图案从底部开始,从深粉色逐渐过渡到浅粉色,在标题"Woman Sure"的上方结束。大约在这个高度,栅格图案的方向从向上变为横向。在栅格图案附近为较深的粉色,在罐子的背面方向逐渐过渡为较浅的粉色。叶子的图案涵盖了各种粉色,采用从小到大的尺寸进行印刷。

此外,该罐的创新之处在于它的容量——125 mL 的容量相当于 250 mL 的喷雾罐体。这意味着不仅减少了材料的使用,而且在保持雅致外观的同时,最大限度地减少了罐体的重量和运输成本。

2014-1 号罐 360 度旋转视频二维码

编号:2014-2

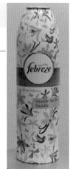

英文介绍

Can No. 2: Febreze "Vanilla"

Marketed Can

Description: The Febreze "Vanilla" can is a striking example of a collaboration between the content and the print design of the can. The design shows the vanilla blossom and the vanilla bean in harmony with birds and dragonflys. The fine and fragile yet clear and detailed stems of the flowers add lightness and vibrance to this can like a breeze. Close-ups show the details of the print are remarkable: the two colours of the body of the dragonfly and its antennae show the craftsmanship of printing. The tiny details are very clear and always on the spot. Also the birds show off very fine details in its wings.

中文介绍

2 号罐:

已上市罐

产品说明:

风倍清的"香草"罐是内容物与印刷设计完美结合的典范。设计展现了香草花、香草豆和鸟儿、蜻蜓和谐共处的画面。花朵细而脆弱,但线条清晰,细节鲜明,仿佛一阵微风为罐装产品增添了轻盈与活力。近距离观察,可以看到蜻蜓翅膀上的两种颜色及其触须的印刷工艺,细节清晰,恰到好处。鸟儿的翅膀也展现出非常精致的细节。

2014-2 号罐 360 度旋转视频二维码

编号：2014-3

Can No. 3: Dove

Marketed Can

Description: Dove—a clean fresh look for a deodorant. The photorealistic image of a pomegranate with the very fine degrading of the kernels add to this clean and fresh image the can displays. But the real innovation is the size and its corresponding content in this curvy shaped can. The can is filled with a deo concentrate that will last as long as a 250 mL can. This means saving material, weight and transport cost and having the same amount as 250 mL for us only in a 125 mL can.

3 号罐：

已上市罐

产品说明：

多芬是一款清新爽洁的香体剂罐。逼真的石榴图像、石榴籽的细致渐变，为这款清新爽洁的产品增添了亮点。然而，真正的创新在于这个独特的弧形容器的大小和相应的内容物。它装有浓缩的香体剂，其使用时间相当于 250 mL 罐子。这意味着可以节省材料、减轻重量、降低运输成本，而我们只需用 125 mL 的罐子提供相当于 250 mL 使用时间的产品。

2014-3 号罐 360 度旋转视频二维码

编号：2014-4

Can No. 4: Neutrogena Beach Defense

Marketed Can

Description: The attractive twin rings on the top sidewall of this container not only add a pleasing look that sets it apart from its competitors on the shelf, but also provide an easy grip that will resist slipping during use. The sunny graphics of this container add to the light airy feel of the container design.

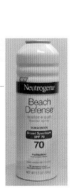

中 文 介 绍

4 号罐：

已上市罐

产品说明：

这个容器顶部引人注目的双环不仅使其在货架上与竞争对手区别开来，而且能提供在使用时易于抓握的防滑功能。罐体上充满活力的图案增加了设计的轻盈感。

2014-4 号罐 360 度旋转视频二维码

编号：2014-5

英 文 介 绍

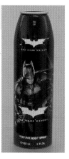

Can No. 5: The Dark Knight

Marketed Can

Description: The Dark Knight, 45 mm × 150 mm, bullet shoulder can, white basecoat, four process colours plus specials, glossy overvarnish.

中 文 介 绍

5 号罐：

已上市罐

产品说明：

该款罐体印有黑暗骑士形象，45 mm×150 mm，具有子弹形肩、白色底涂层、四种基础色以及特殊的光油。

2014-5 号罐 360 度旋转视频二维码

编号：2014-6

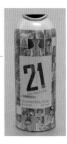

英 文 介 绍

Can No. 6: 21st Generation Female
Marketed Can

Description: 21st Generation Female, 53 mm×140 mm, round shoulder can, transparent basecoat, four process colours plus specials, glossy overvarnish.

中 文 介 绍

6 号罐：

已上市罐

产品说明：

该款罐体是 21 世纪现代女性款，53 mm×140 mm，圆肩、透明底涂层、四种基础色以及特殊的光油。

2014-6 号罐 360 度旋转视频二维码

编号：2014-7

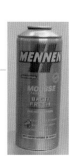

英 文 介 绍

Can No. 7: L'Oréal Mennen Shaving Foam
Marketed Can

Description: The producer's aluminium transfer cans range combines the strengths of both monobloc cans and 3-piece tinplate cans. The producer has met the challenge to develop the first aluminium transfer can in diameter 57 mm to allow L'Oréal to switch from tinplate to aluminium aerosol cans for mennen shaving foam. Forming and delivering a robust flat shoulder with a rim compatible with spraycaps and actuators of tinplate cans on such a big diameter is a market first, now allowing designers to take the advantage of the premium seamless brushed aluminium background to create outstanding artworks.

中 文 介 绍

7 号罐：

已上市罐

产品说明：

该款铝改良铝罐系列由单体罐和三片马口铁罐的优点组合而成。生产商成功开发出有史以来第一个直径为 57 mm 的铝罐，使欧莱雅能够将男士剃须泡沫的包装从马口铁罐转换到铝制喷雾罐。在如此大的直径的罐体上形成并提供坚固的平肩,其边缘与马口铁罐的喷嘴帽和活塞相兼容,这是市场上的首创,使设计师可利用优质无缝抛光铝背景来创造这种非凡的作品。

2014-7号罐360度旋转视频二维码

编号:2014-8

英文介绍

Can No. 8: Sapeco- Laboratoires Venus

Marketed Can

Description: These cans introduce a fresh look consumer can feel! The touch effect newly developed by the producer significantly increases interaction opportunities with consumer who can use two senses instead of just one. These cans developed for Laboratoires Venus improve both ergonomics with embossed grips and feel with a tactile effect on the side, combining two innovations on one can.

中文介绍

8号罐:

已上市罐

产品说明:

该系列罐为消费者带来了全新的视觉体验。生产商新开发的触觉效果显著增加了消费者与产品的互动机会,消费者可以通过两种感官(视觉和触觉)来体验产品,这些罐体由萨佩科-劳伦蒂斯维纳斯特别设计的罐子,不仅提高了罐子的握持舒适度,还在罐身增加了触觉效果,在一个罐体上融合了两项创新。

2014-8号罐360度旋转视频二维码

编号:2014-9

英文介绍

Can No. 9: Système U deo Range

Prototypes Can

Description: These days when you have to choose between a matte or a glossy can are over! The producer now offers a new printing technology that enables you to combine matte and gloss finishes on the same can, creating areas with different look and feel. This new printing process allows you to choose the finish of each colour and creates a look that consumers can touch as well as see, enhancing shelf appeal and product interaction. A first example with the mock ups proposed by the producer to enhance Système U deo range, highlighting some parts of the artwork.

中文介绍

9号罐:

样品罐

产品说明:

消费者不得不在哑光罐或亮光罐之间做出选择的日子已经结束! 目前生产商提供了一种新的印刷技术,可以在同一罐体上结合哑光和亮光两种表面处理,从而呈现出不同的视觉和触觉效果。这种创新的印刷工艺可以让您能够选择各种颜色的油墨,并创造出消费者可以看到和触摸到的外观,从而提升产品在货架上的吸引力和产品互动性。生产商提供的第一个例子是为 Systeme U 化妆品系列设计的样品,以突出其艺术效果的某些部分。

2014-9 号罐 360 度旋转视频二维码

十二、2013年国际铝气雾罐竞赛参赛罐

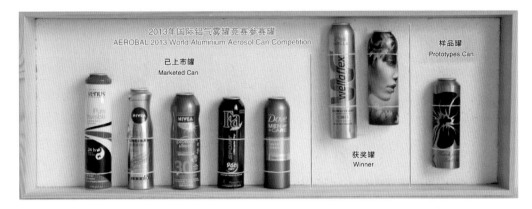

罐编号从左至右分别是:7,2,5,8,1,3,4,6

编号:2013-1

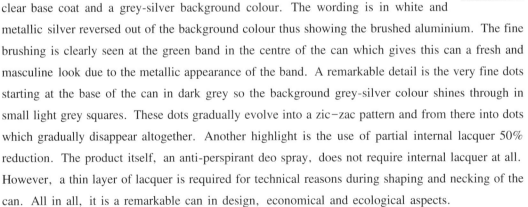

英文介绍

Can No. 1: Dove Men + Care

Marketed Can

Description: Dove Men + Care is a can that offers excellent print design and an eco-logical and economical approach regarding the use of internal lacquer. The can has a clear base coat and a grey-silver background colour. The wording is in white and metallic silver reversed out of the background colour thus showing the brushed aluminium. The fine brushing is clearly seen at the green band in the centre of the can which gives this can a fresh and masculine look due to the metallic appearance of the band. A remarkable detail is the very fine dots starting at the base of the can in dark grey so the background grey-silver colour shines through in small light grey squares. These dots gradually evolve into a zic-zac pattern and from there into dots which gradually disappear altogether. Another highlight is the use of partial internal lacquer 50% reduction. The product itself, an anti-perspirant deo spray, does not require internal lacquer at all. However, a thin layer of lacquer is required for technical reasons during shaping and necking of the can. All in all, it is a remarkable can in design, economical and ecological aspects.

中文介绍

1号罐:

已上市罐

产品说明:

　　该款是多芬男士护理用品,具有独特的印刷设计,在内部涂层的使用方面采用环保和经济的方法。该罐具有透明的底涂层,背景色为银灰色,而文字则以白色和金属银呈现,从背景颜色中反向印出,从而显示出磨砂铝的效果。值得注意的是,由于金属外观的条纹,罐体中心的绿色带经过精细刷涂,增添了清新和阳刚的感觉。一个显著的细节是从罐体底部开始的非常精细的深灰色圆点,让小的浅灰色方块显示出底层的银灰色。这些点逐渐转变成锯齿状,然后逐渐消失不见。另一个值得注意的方面是内部涂层的使用减少了50%。虽然这种防汗香体喷雾罐不需要任何内部涂层,但出于技术原因,在罐的成型和缩颈加工过程中,仍需涂刷一层薄薄的涂层。总的来说,该罐在设计、经济和生态方面都表现出色。

2013-1 号罐 360 度旋转视频二维码

编号:2013-2

英文介绍

Can No. 2: Nivea-Styling Mousse

Marketed Can

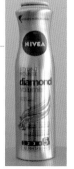

Description: This is a can with an extreme shape. And it shows excellent craftmanship in terms of printing regarding the brand logo "Nivea". The logo is set and printed in a way so that after shaping and necking of the can the logo appears round, resembling the famous blue container. The innovation of the can is the internal lacquer. In this specific case it is possible to use epoxy powder coating which is solvent free as a substitute for PAM internal lacquer. The substitution is possible—provided the formula of the content is suitable for epoxy powder internal lacquer.

中文介绍

2 号罐:

已上市罐

产品说明:

　　这是一个极具创意的罐子形状。在品牌标志"Nivea"印刷上展示了非凡的工艺。罐体经过塑形和缩颈后,该标识看起来是圆形的,类似于标志性的蓝色容器。该罐的创新之处在于其内部涂层。在这种特定情况下,只要罐内产品的配方适合环氧树脂粉末涂层,使用无溶剂的环氧粉末涂层来替代 PAM 内部涂层是可行的。

2013-2 号罐 360 度旋转视频二维码

编号：2013-3

英文介绍

Can No. 3: Wellaflex

Marketed Can

Description: This can attracts the sophisticated buyer with purchasing power at the first moment of truth on the shelf. The embossing around the big letters "WF" has been interrupted in the middle to allow smooth space for printing the wording "wellaflex" on top. The print and embossing is perfectly aligned and makes this a visual and haptical experience. The manufacturer configured the production line in such a way that the speed of production is not altered compared to a can without embossing. This is a truly special aluminium can with a distinguished look and appearance.

中文介绍

3 号罐：

已上市罐

产品说明：

这款罐体在货架上第一时间就能吸引具有购买力的高端消费者。"WF"大写字母周围的浮雕在中间被打断，以便在顶部留出平滑的空间来印刷"wellaflex"的字样。印刷和浮雕完美对齐，从而在视觉和触觉上给人带来愉悦的体验。生产商确保采用浮雕罐印刷不会影响生产速度。这是一款外貌与外表都与众不同的铝制罐。

2013-3 号罐 360 度旋转视频二维码

编号:2013-4

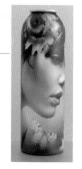

英文介绍

Can No. 4: Autumn

Prototypes Can

Description: This can is an example what state of the art printing systems and complementary colours are capable of. The company HINTERKOPF has provided the digital print. A magnificent print with a fotorealistic image of a woman's face where the extremely fine degrading is well shown on the cheek bones and on the back ground of the can design. The oak leaves provide a powerful contrast to the intensive black hair. The amazing can is proof what new exiting possibilities lie ahead in terms of printing.

中文介绍

4 号罐:

样品罐

产品说明:

　　该罐体是现代印刷系统和配套颜色所能达到的先进水平的典范。由 HINTERKOPF 公司提供数字印刷服务。展示了一个逼真的女性面部图像,特别是在颧骨处和背景设计上清晰地显示了极其细腻的渐变效果。橡树叶与浓密的黑发形成了鲜明的对比。这一非凡的罐体证明了印刷技术中蕴藏着令人兴奋的新的可能性。

2013-4 号罐 360 度旋转视频二维码

编号:2013-5

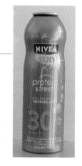

英文介绍

Can No. 5: Nivea Sun Protect & Fresh (200 mL)

Marketed Can

Description: This is a tailormade aluminium packaging which has been developed in cooperation with the client. The ergonomical shape guarantees simple handling of the product and moreover the shape adopts and focuses excellently the logo. The metallic background looks classy and communicates coolness and elegance. Both elements make a great visual and functional impression. The 6-colour print decor submits freshness and naturalness. Summarizing one can say this aerosol can combines perfectly optical, tactile and haptical qualities and therefore is the optimal packaging for a practical application of sun-care products.

中 文 介 绍

5 号罐：

已上市罐

产品说明：

　　这是一款专为客户定制的铝制包装。符合人体工程学的形状确保产品易于抓握,并有效地突出了品牌标志。金属色的背景散发出精致的气息,传达出一种凉爽和优雅的感觉。这两个元素共同营造出视觉和功能上的良好印象。六色印刷装饰赋予产品清新自然的感觉。总之,这种气雾剂罐可以完美地结合视觉、触觉和抓握感品质,使其成为防晒产品的一个理想包装。

2013-5 号罐 360 度旋转视频二维码

编号：2013-6

英 文 介 绍

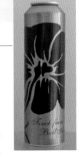

Can No. 6: Tactile Can

Prototypes Can

Description: The producer has been working for many years with suppliers on printing techniques and raw materials, in view to manufacture cans that are providing the most advantages to customers. It is particularly the case for this aerosol can to show a tactile effect. The aim is to customize the can taking advantages for the customer regarding the printing effect with a nice relief and shiny effect depending of the light. It is an opportunity against counterfeiting. This tactile effect creates a guarantee for the consumer as well.

中 文 介 绍

6 号罐：

样品罐

产品说明：

　　多年来生产商一直与供应商在印刷技术和原材料方面合作,以期为客户生产出最具优势的罐子。这种气雾剂罐具有独特的触觉效果,其目的是利用印刷效果来为客户定制罐子,使其在光线照射下呈现出美观的浮雕和光泽效果。这不仅起到了防伪的作用,这种触感效果也为消费者提供了保障。

2013-6 号罐 360 度旋转视频二维码

编号：2013-7

英 文 介 绍

Can No. 7: Laboratoires Venus Pure Invisible Deodorant(200 mL)

Marketed Can

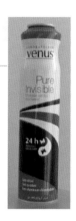

Description: The producer has been working for many years with suppliers on printing techniques and raw materials, with a very close collaboration with his customers in view to manufacture cans that are providing the most advantages to customers. It has been particularly the case for this aerosol can with a tactile effect to secure the market against counterfeiting. This tactile effect provides a guarantee for the consumer.

中 文 介 绍

7 号罐：

已上市罐

产品说明：

多年来生产商一直与供应商在印刷技术和原材料方面密切合作，以满足客户的需求，生产出能够为客户带来最大利益的罐装产品。特别是这种具有触觉效果的气雾罐，旨在防止假冒产品进入市场。这种触感效果为消费者提供了保证。

2013-7 号罐 360 度旋转视频二维码

编号：2013-8

英 文 介 绍

Can No. 8: FA Sport Ultimate Dry

Marketed Can

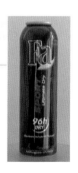

Description: The producers have developed, thanks to their process ability and knows how through the whole supply chain, a new monobloc aluminum can in 150

mL can size. They have successfully managed to lead the aluminium can development FA Sport Ultimate Dry for one of their key customers in Germany: Henkel. The innovation is the first can using the new Ball Recycled Aluminum slugs "ReAl" and the world's first lighter weight industrial aluminium can with recycled material. Indeed the Ball ReAl 25 technology allows Henkel FA Sport Ultimate Dry aerosol can to improve significantly their sustainability impact using 10% less aluminium for the same aerosol can performance.

中文介绍

8 号罐：

已上市罐

产品说明：

生产商已经成功地开发了一种全新的单体铝罐,容量为 150 毫升,这要归功于他们对整个供应链中工艺能力和专业知识的了解。他们成功地为德国的主要客户之一汉高开发了能引领铝罐的发展趋势的 FA 运动干爽气雾铝罐。这款罐体不仅是第一个使用 Ball 的 ReAl 技术的突破性创新,也是世界上第一个使用回收材料的轻量化的工业铝罐。事实上,Ball ReAl 25 技术使得汉高的 FA 运动干爽气雾剂罐可以在保持最佳性能的同时减少 10% 的铝用量,从而显著提升了其可持续性影响。

2013-8 号罐 360 度旋转视频二维码

十三、2012 年国际铝气雾罐竞赛参赛罐

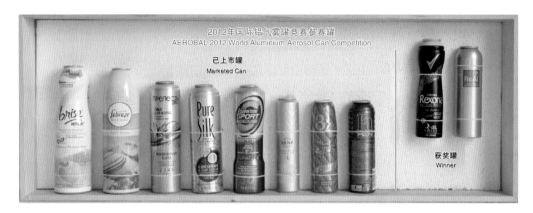

罐编号从左至右分别是:11,3,10,9,1,7,5,8,4,2

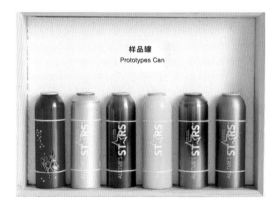

罐编号从左至右分别是:6,12-1,12-2,12-3,12-4,12-5

编号:2012-1

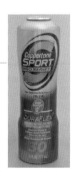

英 文 介 绍

Can No. 1: Coppertone Sport

Marketed Can

Description: CCL Container has expanded its shaping capabilities to now include all geography from the top of the can down to virtually the can bottom. CCL Container's full body shaping technology allows marketers to create unique eye catching packages as evidenced in the Coppertone Sport Pro Series Continuous Spray line marketed by Merck.

1 号罐：

已上市罐

产品说明：

CCL 公司已将其成型能力扩展到了从罐顶到几乎罐底的所有区域。CCL 公司的全罐身成型技术使营销人员能够创造出独特的引人注目的包装，这在由 Merck 公司推广的 Coppertone Sport Pro 系列喷雾产品上得到了体现。

2012-1 号罐 360 度旋转视频二维码

编号：2012-2

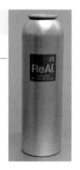

Can No. 2: ReAl™

Prototypes Can

Description: The presented aerosol can named ReAl™ can is the world's first lightweight aluminium aerosol can containing 25 percent of recycled aluminium. This metal technology breakthrough enables the use of recycled aluminium in the manufacture of extruded aluminium packaging for aerosols. The resulting new metal alloy exhibits increased strength and allows to lighten the container by as much as 10 percent without affecting package integrity. ReAl™ brand cans will improve the carbon footprint of increasingly popular extruded aluminium packaging by enabling to reduce the amount of metal in the package and further enhance the environmental performance of Ball Aerocan.

2 号罐：

样品罐

产品说明：

这款名为 ReAlTM 的气雾剂罐是全球首款轻型铝气雾剂罐，含有 25% 的回收铝。这项金属技术的突破使回收铝能够用于挤压成型铝制气雾罐。由此产生的新型金属合金具有更高的强度，并允许在不影响包装完整性的情况下减轻多达 10% 的重量。ReAlTM 品牌气雾罐将通过减少包装中的金属含量，改善日益流行的挤压铝包装的碳足迹，从而进一步提高 Ball 气雾罐的环保性能。

2012-2 号罐 360 度旋转视频二维码

编号：**2012-3**

英文介绍

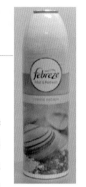

Can No. 3: Febreze Coastal Escape

Marketed Can

Description: This can impresses with its bullet shape. The flange shows a 15-degree angle in order to guarantee perfect closeness. The design, which is created with 8 colours, is achieved by an ink separation device and applying a white base coat. In the foreground of the print design a shell is clearly and perfectly visible and acts as an eye catcher because of its photorealistic look. The background is out of focus, giving the impression of being at the bottom of the sea. The top of the can has a fine degrading print in various shades of blue. To complete the clean and refreshing look a glossy overcoat is applied. All in all, the print design and the content go extremely well together, because this can gives the buyer the feeling of inhaling a fresh breeze at the sea shore.

中文介绍

3 号罐：

已上市罐

产品说明：

这款罐子以其子弹形设计令人印象深刻。罐体凸缘呈 15°角，确保罐体具有可靠的密封性能。这个由 8 种颜色组成的设计是通过分色技术和白色底涂层实现的。在印刷设计的主视面中，一个贝壳清晰而完美地呈现，并因其逼真的外观而引人注目。罐体背景被虚化，给人一种置身海底的感觉。罐体的顶部印有多种蓝色渐变图案，精细而优雅。为了达到清晰和清爽的外观效果，罐体表面涂有一层高光油。总而言之，印刷设计和内容完美契合，它让消费者感受到了一种在海边呼吸清新微风的感觉。

2012-3 号罐 360 度旋转视频二维码

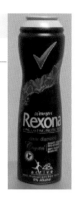

编号：2012-4

英 文 介 绍

Can No. 4: Rexona Clear Diamond

Marketed Can

Description: This can has a very feminine and distinctive shape. The black print and the lavender lace give this can an elegant look. The brushed aluminium shines through the lavender of the lace giving it a three dimensional look. The logo on the upper part of the can captivates the eye with the fine degrading of the purple colour and the fine contour in brushed aluminium. A further highlight is the negative print of the brand name, which is striking but suits this classical design perfectly. The matt overvarnish completes the design.

中 文 介 绍

4 号罐：

已上市罐

产品说明：

　　这款罐体拥有一个非常女性化和独特的形状。黑色印花和淡紫色蕾丝赋予罐子优雅的外观。蕾丝上的淡紫色与磨砂铝的光泽相得益彰，呈现出立体感。罐体顶部的品牌标志以磨砂铝的精细轮廓和精细的紫色渐变而吸引眼球。罐体的另一个亮点是品牌名称的负片印刷，非常显目，与这种经典的设计完美搭配。哑光设计则为整个设计画上了完美的句号。

2012-4 号罐 360 度旋转视频二维码

编号：2012-5

英 文 介 绍

Can No. 5: Glam Up 8×4

Marketed Can

Description: This can with its pink and silver design and its distinctive finely conical shape is a real eye catcher on the shelf and has a high recognition value. The print design with its fine degrading colours resembles an haute couture handbag. The brand name in brushed aluminium has a beautifully glow. The bracelet which is printed in silver with the sparkling lucky charms gives the impression of being real. The fine vignetted halftone of the emblem further enhances the posh impression. A glossy overcoat completes the glamorous design. This stylish can comes with an ecological friendly internal powder coating, which is solvent free.

中文介绍

5 号罐:

已上市罐

产品说明:

　　该款罐采用粉色和银色设计,外观呈独特的细锥形,在货架上非常引人注目,具有很高的辨识度。其印刷设计采用渐变色印花,看起来像一件高级定制手提包。抛光铝罐上的品牌名称在灯光下闪闪发光。印刷的银色手镯上印着闪闪发光的幸运符,给人一种逼真的感觉。徽章的精致晕染色调使得罐体更高雅。闪亮的光油使这个迷人的设计更加完美。这款时尚的罐体内有一层环保的无溶剂粉末涂层。

2012-5 号罐 360 度旋转视频二维码

编号:**2012-6**

英文介绍

Can No. 6: The Star-Money

Prototypes Can

Description: The design of the can shows the fairy tale "*The Star-Money*". The dark blue print resembles the night. The fairy tale figure is printed in black with its highlights being accentuated by the brushed aluminium. In order to give a visual and also

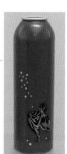

haptical effect, metallic stars are applied which give this design the impression of sparkling stars falling from heaven.

中文介绍

6 号罐:

样品罐

产品说明:

　　这款罐体的设计源于童话故事《星币》(The Star-Money)。深蓝色的印花衬托着夜色。童话人物用黑色印刷,通过磨砂铝突出其亮点。为了达到一种视觉和触觉兼具的效果,罐体上设计了金属星星,给人一种闪闪发光的星星从天而降的感觉。

2012-6 号罐 360 度旋转视频二维码

编号：2012-7

Can No. 7: Molt Bene, Bene Color Shine Whip Cream

Marketed Can

Description: Three factors are in one can:

1) Barrier pack (we call it TUB system) assembles a plastic bag into the can. Fill propellant gas into the gap between can and bag. When content comes out without gas mixing, we will get whip cream like product.

2) Surface shaping with printing process. Without using additional facility, surface shaping is available by usual printing process. Less investment required.

3) Hot stamp. Putting thicker film than standard hot stamp. It can make more gorgeous effect for surface decoration.

7 号罐：

已上市罐

产品说明：

这个罐体包含三个要素：

1）屏障包装（我们称之为 TUB 系统）。将一个塑料袋装入罐体里。将推进剂气体填充到罐体和袋子之间的空隙中。这样当内容物流出时，不会与气体混合，我们就会得到奶油霜一样的产品。

2）采用表面成型的印刷工艺。无需额外的设备即可通过常规的印刷工艺实现表面成型。需要的投资较少。

3）烫印。使用比标准烫印更厚的膜可以使表面装饰更加华丽。

2012-7 号罐 360 度旋转视频二维码

编号:2012-8

Can No. 8: FA Men Xtreme Dry

Marketed Can

Description: The producer has successfully managed to lead the aluminium can development, the full industrialization and finally the full supply of this new product FA Men Xtreme Dry, for one of his customers in Germany: Henkel. The innovation resides in the visual effect created by the combination of embossed—Debossed body shape and the corresponding printed design. The final result is a new elegant aluminium monobloc can, in diameter 45 mm, keeping a customised can design characteristics linked to an original feature. The embossed—Debossed can body shape design, reinforces the product performance spirit.

中 文 介 绍

8 号罐:

已上市罐

产品说明:

生产商成功地引领铝罐工业化进程,并最终为其德国客户之一汉高提供了这款新产品 FA 男士干爽气雾剂罐。其创新之处在于将凹凸造型与相应的印刷设计相结合所产生的视觉效果。最终制成一款直径 45 mm 新的优雅的铝制单体罐,保留了与原始特征相关的定制罐的设计特性。凹凸造型设计强化了产品的性能。

2012-8 号罐 360 度旋转视频二维码

编号:2012-9

中 文 介 绍

Can No. 9: Pure Silk

Marketed Can

Description: The Pure Silk container is printed using a combination of four color process and match color on a brushed aluminum monobloc aerosol container with a gloss exterior varnish. This can has an eco-gorge shoulder with a one inch outside curl.

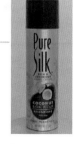

中 文 介 绍

9 号罐:

已上市罐

产品说明：

Pure Silk 产品使用四色工艺和配色的组合印刷,在抛光铝单体气雾罐的外层涂有光油。该罐拥有一个对环保友好的肩部设计,肩部外侧带有一英寸的卷边口径。

2012-9 号罐 360 度旋转视频二维码

编号：2012-10

英 文 介 绍

Can No. 10: PRELEST

Marketed Can

Description: This aluminium can has been designed and put into production in 2012.

It is made due to the recent development approaches in can manufacturing sphere:

New format-diameter 50 mm.

Can be combined with spray cap.

The can has very modern and simple design with brushing effect.

"PRELEST" is the own brand name of the producer.

Nobody in Russia and CIS produces such format of the can by now.

中 文 介 绍

10 号罐:

已上市罐

产品说明:

该铝罐已于 2012 年设计并投入生产。

它是根据当前易拉罐生产领域的最新发展理念制造的:

新规格直径为 50 mm。

可与喷雾盖配合使用。

易拉罐设计现代简约,带有磨砂效果。

"PRELEST"是生产商的自有品牌。

目前,俄罗斯和独联体还没有生产这种规格的罐子。

2012-10 号罐 360 度旋转视频二维码

编号：**2012-11**

英 文 介 绍

Can No. 11: Brise Refresh Fraîcheur Pomme Verte

Marketed Can

Description: The Glade/Brise cans as presented for SC Johnson feature two innovative aspects of aluminium impact extruded can making.

Long stroke, extreme shaping. The ratio between the original extrusion diameter and the diameter reduction as achieved during the process of producing the Glade/Brise cans is approaching the extremes of what is industrially possible within the impact extrusion process.

Hi def, Full colour printing. The producer's use of its capability to print full colour/CMYK on aluminium cans is an industry first and is used on the Glade/Brise cans with dry offset printing machines. This capability opens a wide range of printing possibilities previously not possible due to restrictions of Pantone referenced colours/printing and/or available number of ink containers on printing units.

中 文 介 绍

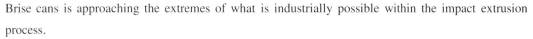

11 号罐：

已上市罐

产品说明：

庄臣公司（SC Johnson）推出的铝制冲压罐具有两项创新的冲压罐制造技术。长冲程和极限成型。Glade/Brise 罐生产过程中原始冲压直径与直径减小之间的比率接近在工业上冲击挤压工艺可能达到的极限。高清晰度，全彩印刷。生产商在铝罐上印刷全彩/CMYK 图案是行业首创，并使用干式胶印机在 Glade/Brise 罐上打印。这一功能开辟了广泛印刷的可能性，以前受潘通参考颜色/印刷限制/印刷单元中可用墨盒数量的限制而无法实现。

2012-11 号罐 360 度旋转视频二维码

编号：2012-12-1

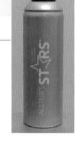

Can No. 12-1: Alltub's Stars[Glittering Effect (Gray)]

Prototypes Can

Description: It represents a prestigious technical project for Alltub, unique for its customers and designed in particular for premium cosmetic products. Alltub's aim is to change the final aspect of cans and find out new solutions, similar to the packaging of high perfumery products (glass for perfumes and make-up holders). Thanks to these effects, cans will be very similar to the packaging of the highest standard for new market challenges, reaching levels not possible with traditional production technology.

You have been sent cans representing five of the various effects tested by Alltub and presented to our customers. They are part of a complete range of eye-catchers that boost the visual impact of aluminium cans.

Glittering effect(gray): On this can is applied a silver glittering varnish containing very big metallic particles, that our traditional technology can not normally apply in equal measure all over the can surface.

Droplet effect(purple): This can is made "fresh" by realistic water droplets all over the can surface, giving a wet look ideal for the cosmetic market.

Pearled shaded effect(green): On this can is applied a shaded, pearled, transparent varnish in equal measure on the overall surface.

Iridescent(black) and many-coloured paillette(blue) effect: This can offers an astonishing colour effect with innumerable shades. The resulting optical effects are harmonious and dazzling.

中 文 介 绍

12-1 号罐：

样品罐

产品说明：

它代表了 Alltub 的一个著名技术项目,对于客户来说是独一无二的,专为高端化妆品而设计。Alltub 的目标是改变罐体的最终外观,并找到新的解决方案,类似于高档香水产品的包装(香水和化妆品用玻璃瓶)。由于这些效果,罐体将非常接近最高标准的包装,以应对新的市场挑战,达到传统生产技术无法达到的水平。

我们已将 Alltub 测试的五种不同效果的罐体发送给客户。它们是一系列引人注目的罐体的一部分,大大提升了铝罐的视觉冲击力。

闪耀效果(灰色):在这个罐体上使用一种含有非常大金属颗粒的银色光油,这是我们传统的技术无法做到的。

水滴效果(紫色):在罐体表面模拟出逼真的水滴效果,赋予其湿润的外观,非常适合化妆品市场。

珍珠光泽(绿色):在整个罐体表面均匀地涂覆珠光光油。

变幻莫测的(黑色)和多彩调色板(蓝色)效果:这两款罐体提供了令人惊叹的色彩效果,拥有无数种色调。最终的光学效果和谐而耀眼。

2012-12-1号罐360度旋转视频二维码

编号:2012-12-2

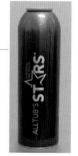

英文介绍

Can No. 12-2: Alltub's Stars[Droplet Effect(Purple)]

Prototypes Can

Description: It represents a prestigious technical project for Alltub, unique for its customers and designed in particular for premium cosmetic products. Alltub's aim is to change the final aspect of cans and find out new solutions, similar to the packaging of high perfumery products (glass for perfumes and make-up holders). Thanks to these effects, cans will be very similar to the packaging of the highest standard for new market challenges, reaching levels not possible with traditional production technology.

You have been sent cans representing five of the various effects tested by Alltub and presented to our customers. They are part of a complete range of eye-catchers that boost the visual impact of aluminium cans.

Glittering effect(gray): On this can is applied a silver glittering varnish containing very big metallic particles, that our traditional technology can not normally apply in equal measure all over the can surface.

Droplet effect(purple): This can is made "fresh" by realistic water droplets all over the can surface, giving a wet look ideal for the cosmetic market.

Pearled shaded effect(green): On this can is applied a shaded, pearled, transparent varnish in equal measure on the overall surface.

Iridescent(black) and many-coloured paillette(blue) effect: This can offers an astonishing colour effect with innumerable shades. The resulting optical effects are harmonious and dazzling.

中文介绍

12-2号罐:

样品罐

产品说明:

它代表了Alltub的一个著名技术项目,对于客户来说是独一无二的,专为高端化妆品而设计。Alltub 的目标是改变罐体的最终外观,并找到新的解决方案,类似于高档香水产品的包装(香水和化妆品用玻璃瓶)。由于这些效果,罐体将非常接近最高标准的包装,以应对新的市场挑战,达到传统生产技术无法达到的水平。

我们已将 Alltub 测试的五种不同效果的罐体发送给客户。它们是一系列引人注目的罐体的一部分,大大提升了铝罐的视觉冲击力。

闪耀效果(灰色):在这个罐体上使用一种含有非常大金属颗粒的银色光油,这是我们传统的技术无法做到的。

水滴效果(紫色):在罐体表面模拟出逼真的水滴效果,赋予其湿润的外观,非常适合化妆品市场。

珍珠光泽(绿色):在整个罐体表面均匀地涂覆珠光光油。

变幻莫测的(黑色)和多彩调色板(蓝色)效果:这两款罐体提供了令人惊叹的色彩效果,拥有无数种色调。最终的光学效果和谐而耀眼。

2012-12-2 号罐 360 度旋转视频二维码

编号:**2012-12-3**

英文介绍————————————————————

Can No.12-3: Alltub's Stars[Rearled Shaded Effect (green)]

Prototypes Can

Description: It represents a prestigious technical project for Alltub, unique for its customers and designed in particular for premium cosmetic products. Alltub's aim is to change the final aspect of cans and find out new solutions, similar to the packaging of high perfumery products (glass for perfumes and make-up holders). Thanks to these effects, cans will be very similar to the packaging of the highest standard for new market challenges, reaching levels not possible with traditional production technology.

You have been sent cans representing five of the various effects tested by Alltub and presented to our customers. They are part of a complete range of eye-catchers that boost the visual impact of aluminium cans.

Glittering effect(gray): On this can is applied a silver glittering varnish containing very big metallic particles, that our traditional technology can not normally apply in equal measure all over the can surface.

Droplet effect(purple): This can is made "fresh" by realistic water droplets all over the can surface, giving a wet look ideal for the cosmetic market.

Pearled shaded effect(green): On this can is applied a shaded, pearled, transparent varnish in equal measure on the overall surface.

Iridescent(black) and many-coloured paillette(blue) effect: This can offers an astonishing colour effect with innumerable shades. The resulting optical effects are harmonious and dazzling.

中文介绍

12-3 号罐：

样品罐

产品说明：

它代表了 Alltub 的一个著名技术项目,对于客户来说是独一无二的,专为高端化妆品而设计。Alltub 的目标是改变罐体的最终外观,并找到新的解决方案,类似于高档香水产品的包装(香水和化妆品用玻璃瓶)。由于这些效果,罐体将非常接近最高标准的包装,以应对新的市场挑战,达到传统生产技术无法达到的水平。

我们已将 Alltub 测试的五种不同效果的罐体发送给客户。它们是一系列引人注目的罐体的一部分,大大提升了铝罐的视觉冲击力。

闪耀效果(灰色):在这个罐体上使用一种含有非常大金属颗粒的银色光油,这是我们传统的技术无法做到的。

水滴效果(紫色):在罐体表面模拟出逼真的水滴效果,赋予其湿润的外观,非常适合化妆品市场。

珍珠光泽(绿色):在整个罐体表面均匀地涂覆珠光光油。

变幻莫测的(黑色)和多彩调色板(蓝色)效果:这两款罐体提供了令人惊叹的色彩效果,拥有无数种色调。最终的光学效果和谐而耀眼。

2012-12-3 号罐 360 度旋转视频二维码

编号：**2012-12-4**

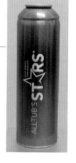

英文介绍

Can No. 12-4: Alltub's Stars[Iridescent Effect(Black)]

Prototypes Can

Description: It represents a prestigious technical project for Alltub, unique for its customers and designed in particular for premium cosmetic products. Alltub's aim is to change the final aspect of cans and find out new solutions, similar to the packaging of high perfumery products (glass for perfumes and make-up holders). Thanks to these effects, cans will be very similar to the packaging of the highest standard for new market challenges, reaching levels not possible with traditional production technology.

You have been sent cans representing five of the various effects tested by Alltub and presented to our customers. They are part of a complete range of eye-catchers that boost the visual impact of aluminium cans.

Glittering effect(gray): On this can is applied a silver glittering varnish containing very big metallic particles, that our traditional technology can not normally apply in equal measure all over the can surface.

Droplet effect(purple): This can is made "fresh" by realistic water droplets all over the can surface, giving a wet look ideal for the cosmetic market.

Pearled shaded effect(green): On this can is applied a shaded, pearled, transparent varnish in equal measure on the overall surface.

Iridescent(black) and many-coloured paillette(blue) effect: This can offers an astonishing colour effect with innumerable shades. The resulting optical effects are harmonious and dazzling.

中文介绍

12-4 号罐：

样品罐

产品说明：

它代表了 Alltub 的一个著名技术项目,对于客户来说是独一无二的,专为高端化妆品而设计。Alltub 的目标是改变罐体的最终外观,并找到新的解决方案,类似于高档香水产品的包装(香水和化妆品用玻璃瓶)。由于这些效果,罐体将非常接近最高标准的包装,以应对新的市场挑战,达到传统生产技术无法达到的水平。

我们已将 Alltub 测试的五种不同效果的罐体发送给客户。它们是一系列引人注目的罐体的一部分,大大提升了铝罐的视觉冲击力。

闪耀效果(灰色):在这个罐体上使用一种含有非常大金属颗粒的银色光油,这是我们传统的技术无法做到的。

水滴效果(紫色):在罐体表面模拟出逼真的水滴效果,赋予其湿润的外观,非常适合化妆品市场。

珍珠光泽(绿色):在整个罐体表面均匀地涂覆珠光光油。

变幻莫测的(黑色)和多彩调色板(蓝色)效果:这两款罐体提供了令人惊叹的色彩效果,拥有无数种色调。最终的光学效果和谐而耀眼。

2012-12-4 号罐 360 度旋转视频二维码

编号:2012-12-5

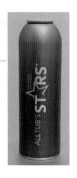

英文介绍

Can No. 12-5: Alltub's Stars[Many-coloured Paillette Effect(Blue)]

Prototypes Can

Description: It represents a prestigious technical project for Alltub, unique for its customers and designed in particular for premium cosmetic products. Alltub's aim is to change the final aspect of cans and find out new solutions, similar to the packaging of high perfumery products (glass for perfumes and make-up holders). Thanks to these effects, cans will be very similar to the packaging of the highest standard for new market challenges, reaching levels not possible with traditional production technology.

You have been sent cans representing five of the various effects tested by Alltub and presented to our customers. They are part of a complete range of eye-catchers that boost the visual impact of aluminium cans.

Glittering effect(gray): On this can is applied a silver glittering varnish containing very big metallic particles, that our traditional technology can not normally apply in equal measure all over the can surface.

Droplet effect(purple): This can is made "fresh" by realistic water droplets all over the can surface, giving a wet look ideal for the cosmetic market.

Pearled shaded effect(green): On this can is applied a shaded, pearled, transparent varnish in equal measure on the overall surface.

Iridescent(black) and many-coloured paillette(blue) effect: This can offers an astonishing colour effect with innumerable shades. The resulting optical effects are harmonious and dazzling.

中文介绍

12-5号罐:

样品罐

产品说明:

它代表了 Alltub 的一个著名技术项目,对于客户来说是独一无二的,专为高端化妆品而设计。Alltub 的目标是改变罐体的最终外观,并找到新的解决方案,类似于高档香水产品的包装(香水和化妆品用玻璃瓶)。由于这些效果,罐体将非常接近最高标准的包装,以应对新的市场挑战,达到传统生产技术无法达到的水平。

我们已将 Alltub 测试的五种不同效果的罐体发送给客户。它们是一系列引人注目的罐体的一部分,大大提升了铝罐的视觉冲击力。

闪耀效果(灰色):在这个罐体上使用一种含有非常大金属颗粒的银色光油,这是我们传统的技术无法做到的。

水滴效果(紫色):在罐体表面模拟出逼真的水滴效果,赋予其湿润的外观,非常适合化妆品市场。

珍珠光泽(绿色):在整个罐体表面均匀地涂覆珠光光油。

变幻莫测的(黑色)和多彩调色板(蓝色)效果:这两款罐体提供了令人惊叹的色彩效果,拥有无数种色调。最终的光学效果和谐而耀眼。

2012-12-5号罐360度旋转视频二维码

十四、2011年国际铝气雾罐竞赛参赛罐

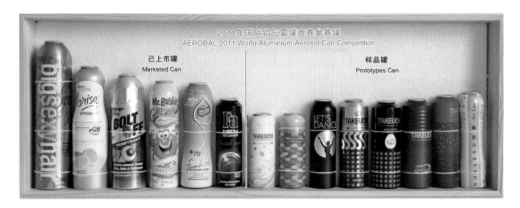

罐编号从左至右分别是:20,12,19,21,1,10,7,7-1,14,5,6,8,9,2

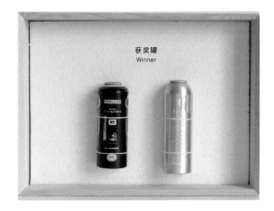

罐编号从左至右分别是:11,4

编号:2011-1

英 文 介 绍

Can No. 1: Evolution Pro(53 mm×175 mm)

Marketed Can

Description: Following the evolution shaped can the technical feasibility has been explored further and we have been successful in realising the stronger and more pronounced waistline of the Evolution Pro Can. The shaped profile gives the aluminium can an attractive and trendy look and it easily fits to hold it. The decoration of the product has been specially applied to respect the distortion (text and illustration) and the background vignette give the design a fresh and clean touch.

中文介绍

1 号罐:

已上市罐

EVOLUTION PRO 53×175 mm

产品说明:

　　随着异型罐技术的进一步成熟,我们已经成功地开发了强度更大、腰线更明显的进化专业型(Evolution Pro)系列罐。这种异型塑造的轮廓使铝罐更具吸引人的时尚外观,且很容易握持。铝罐的印刷经过特殊处理后很好地适应了罐体的变形(文字和插图),其背景的渐变效果使整个设计看起来清新和干净。

2011-1 号罐 360 度旋转视频二维码

编号:2011-2

英文介绍

Can No. 2: Evolution Pro(45 mm×158 mm)

Prototypes Can

Description: In order to expand the Evolution Pro range, a smaller container capable of holding 150 mL of the filled product has been added to this product group. The considerable deformation of the body part of the cylinder gives the aluminium can a very aesthetical look and the overall appearance of the packaging is slim, elaborate and a certain elegant touch cannot be denied.

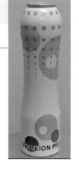

中文介绍

2 号罐:

样品罐

产品说明:

　　为了拓展进化专业型(Evolution Pro)的产品线,该产品系列中增加了一个能够容纳 150 mL 产品的较小容器。罐体部分的显著变形使铝罐具有非常美观的外观,包装的整体外观纤细精致,其整体优雅触感不容忽视。

2011-2 号罐 360 度旋转视频二维码

编号：2011-4

Can No. 4: Brilliant by Nussbaum(50 mm×156 mm)

Prototypes Can

Description: For the first time the hot foil printing is applied as an in-line process. The decoration itself is protected and covered by special glossy over varnish and is therefore resistant to process-related deformation. In the combination with different print methods new opportunities to individually decorated aluminium cans are possible. The vibrancy of the colours are ideal to enhance and strengthen logos and brand names. The shiny colours are suitable to be printed onto different base colours like white, brushed and black.

4 号罐：

样品罐

产品说明：

　　这是首次将热烫印工艺应用于在线生产。印刷图案本身被特殊的光油保护和覆盖,因此具有抗工艺相关的变形。结合不同的印刷方法,在铝罐上分区域印刷成为可能。徽标和品牌名称的颜色饱和度也得到了进一步提高和加强。带有光泽的颜色适合印在白色、磨砂和黑色等不同的底色上。

2011-4 号罐 360 度旋转视频二维码

编号：2011-5

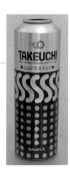

Can No. 5: Emboss Stamped Can

Prototypes Can

Description: Created by printing machine. Perfect registration with artwork available.

5 号罐：

样品罐

产品说明：

　　通过印刷机完成创新,与印刷设计完美匹配。

2011-5 号罐 360 度旋转视频二维码

编号:2011-6

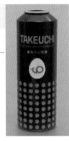

英文介绍

Can No.6: Foaming Ink Can

Prototypes Can

Description: Different touch (smooth and rough) is available on the same surface by using foaming ink.

中文介绍

6 号罐

样品罐

产品说明:

通过使用发泡油墨,可以在同一表面实现不同触感的光滑和粗糙效果。

2011-6 号罐 360 度旋转视频二维码

编号:2011-7

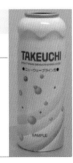

英文介绍

Can No.7: New Wave Line Can

Prototypes Can

Description: Created by conventional necking machine. Unique shape, easy grip.

中文介绍

7 号罐

样品罐

产品说明:

该款罐由常规的缩颈机制造。它具有独特的形状,易于抓握。

2011-7 号罐 360 度旋转视频二维码

编号：**2011-7-1**

英 文 介 绍

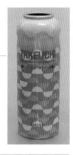

Can No. 7-1: New Wave Line Can

Prototypes Can

Description: Created by conventional necking machine. Unique shape, easy grip.

中 文 介 绍

7-1 号罐

样品罐

产品说明：

　　该款罐由常规的缩颈机制造。它具有独特的形状，易于抓握。

2011-7-1 号罐 360 度旋转视频二维码

编号：**2011-8**

英 文 介 绍

Can No. 8: New Free Form Can

Prototypes Can

Description: Created by conventional necking machine. Unique shape, easy grip.

中 文 介 绍

8 号罐

样品罐

产品说明：

　　该罐由常规的缩颈机制造。它具有独特的形状，更易抓握。

2011-8 号罐 360 度旋转视频二维码

编号：**2011-9**

英 文 介 绍

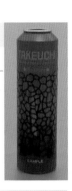

Can No. 9: Brilliant Can

Prototypes Can

Description: High value, gorgeous image appearance available by silk screen printing.

中 文 介 绍

9 号罐

样品罐

产品说明：

采用丝网印刷技术，让罐体上呈现绚丽高价值的图像外观。

2011-9 号罐 360 度旋转视频二维码

编号：**2011-10**

英 文 介 绍

Can No. 10: FA Men Black Sun/FA Men Speedster

Marketed Can

Description: The printing result shows the consequent utilization of the producer's high definition printing for artworks with graphical elements. Being embedded in the black background design of FA's sub brand the visual glares with its full bandwidth of colour gradiations created with 5 colours only. This product packaging attracts the customer's attention directly from the shelf.

中 文 介 绍

10 号罐

已上市罐

产品说明：

　　该印刷效果展示了制造商在图形元素艺术作品上的高清晰度印刷技术的应用。该产品嵌入 FA 子品牌的黑色背景的设计中，仅用 5 种颜色就实现了全色阶的色彩渐变，视觉效果醒目。这款产品包装在货架上就能直接吸引消费者的注意力。

2011-10 号罐 360 度旋转视频二维码

编号：2011-11

英文介绍

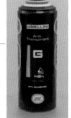

Can No. 11: G. Bellini(200 mL)

Marketed Can

Description: The producer has developed, thanks to his last process ability, a new deep embossed can. He has successfully managed to lead the aluminium can development, the full industrialization and finally the full supply of this new product for one of its customer in Germany: Dalli Win. The innovation resides in the visual effect created by the combination of deep embossed—debossed body shape and the corresponding printed design. The final result is a new elegant aluminium monobloc can, in diameter 53 mm, keeping a customised can design characteristics linked to an original feature. This unique deep embossed—debossed can is not only a technology innovation, but as well a market innovation for the private label business.

中文介绍

11 号罐

已上市罐

产品说明：

　　生产商通过其最新的生产能力开发了一种新型深压纹罐。他成功地引领了铝罐的发展，实现了其产品的全面工业化生产，并最终为德国的一位客户 Dalli Win 提供了这种新产品的全面供应。其创新之处在于深压纹—凹压纹罐体形状与相应印刷设计的结合所产生的视觉效果。最终成果是一款直径 53 mm 的新型的优雅铝制单片罐，保持了与原始特征相关的定制罐的设计特性。这种独特的深压纹—凹压纹罐不仅是一项技术创新，也是自有品牌业务的一项市场创新。

2011-11 号罐 360 度旋转视频二维码

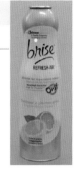

编号：2011-12

英文介绍

Can No. 12: Glade/Brise Refresh-Air

Marketed Can

Description: The aluminium aerosol can is a brand-dedicated shaped aerosol can which is the result of the cooperation between SC Johnson marketing and the producer's technical departments. The can features an ergonomical shape which in combination with the bespoke actuator makes the packaging concept very user-friendly. The producer uses its Hi-def, full-colour printing technology which in combination with the aerosol shape ensures optimal shelf-impact and premium image for this new range of air fresheners.

中文介绍

12 号罐

已上市罐

产品说明：

这款铝质气雾罐是 SC Johnson 营销与生产技术部门合作的成果，是一种专为品牌设计的异形气雾罐。该罐采用人体工学设计，与定制的喷头相结合，由此设计的包装非常便于使用。生产商采用其高保真全彩印刷技术，结合气雾罐形状，确保这款新型空气清新剂在货架上具有最佳视觉冲击力和高端形象。

2011-12 号罐 360 度旋转视频二维码

编号：2011-14

英文介绍

CAN No. 14: Let's Dance

Prototypes Can

Description: The eyecatcher of this elegant mat black printed can is the 3-dimensional dancer that seems to come out of the body of the can. This is achieved by an aluminium coloured, brushed and deeper set background. The writing "Let's Dance" in white letters, brushed embossed aluminium, a dancer that seems to melt with its surrounding, gives the user an immediate optical and haptical feeling of "In this can is my deodorant".

中文介绍
14 号罐
样品罐
产品说明:

　　这款优雅的哑光黑色印花罐最引人注目的地方是一个三维的舞者形象,仿佛要从罐体跃然而出。这是通过对有色的铝的罐体刷上涂料并衬上更深的背景来实现的。白色字母"Let's Dance"(让我们一起跳舞吧),采用抛光铝拉丝浮雕的铝制材料压印,使舞者的形象与周围融为一体,给用户立即有一种"我的香体剂就在此罐中"的视觉和触觉效果。

2011-14 号罐 360 度旋转视频二维码

编号:2011-19

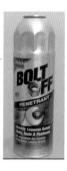

英文介绍
Can No. 19:　Nutek Green Bolt Off Penetrant
Marketed Can
Description: The intricate graphic design of the wrench working on a bolt is further anhanced by the "nuts and bolts" embossed/debossed container shape which provides an easy grip for spraying and eye catching esthetics.

中文介绍
19 号罐
已上市罐
产品说明:

　　通过在螺栓上作业的扳手的复杂图形设计,进一步增强了"螺母和螺栓"压花/凹凸容器形状,便于抓握,同时还具有引人注目的美学效果。

2011-19 号罐 360 度旋转视频二维码

编号：**2011-20**

英文介绍

Can No. 20: Big Sexy Hair Spray & Play

Marketed Can

Description: The beauty of brushed aluminium in combination with tone on tone translucent inks provides a look that will set this product apart on the shelf and promote breast cancer awareness.

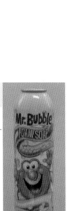

中文介绍

20 号罐

已上市罐

产品说明：

　　拉丝铝喷雾罐的金属光泽与同色调半透明油墨相结合,使得该款产品展现了独特的美感,在货架上格外亮眼,同时也提高了人们对乳腺癌的认识。

2011-20 号罐 360 度旋转视频二维码

编号：**2011-21**

英文介绍

Can No. 21: Mr. Bubble Bubbleberry Foam Soap

Marketed Can

Description: Fun tone on tone graphics combines with a loveable brand recognisable character provides consumer appeal to this happy container.

中文介绍

21 号罐

已上市罐

产品说明：

　　有趣的图案同色融合品牌的可爱的卡通形象,足以吸引消费者对这个充满欢乐的罐的关注。

2011-21 号罐 360 度旋转视频二维码

十五、2009 年国际铝气雾罐竞赛参赛罐

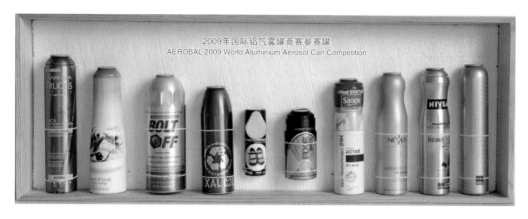

罐编号从左至右分别是：13，16，2，3，10，11，15，1，7，14

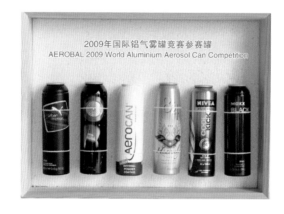

罐编号从左至右分别是：6，8，9，4，12，5

编号：2009-1

2009-1 号罐 360 度旋转视频二维码

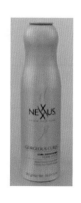

编号：**2009-2**

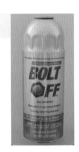

2009-2号罐360度旋转视频二维码

编号：**2009-3**

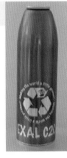

2009-3号罐360度旋转视频二维码

编号：**2009-4**

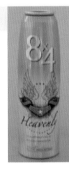

2009-4号罐360度旋转视频二维码

编号：**2009-5**

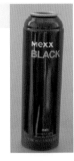

2009-5号罐360度旋转视频二维码

编号：**2009-6**

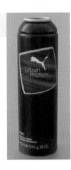

2009-6号罐360度旋转视频二维码

编号：**2009-7**

2009-7 号罐 360 度旋转视频二维码

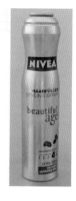

编号：**2009-8**

2009-8 号罐 360 度旋转视频二维码

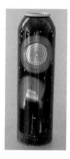

编号：**2009-9**

2009-9 号罐 360 度旋转视频二维码

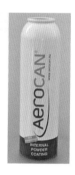

编号：**2009-10**

2009-10 号罐 360 度旋转视频二维码

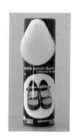

编号：2009-11

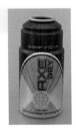

2009-11 号罐 360 度旋转视频二维码

编号：2009-12

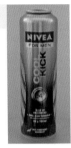

2009-12 号罐 360 度旋转视频二维码

编号：2009-13

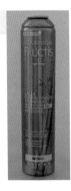

2009-13 号罐 360 度旋转视频二维码

编号：2009-14

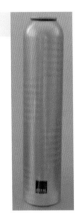

2009-14 号罐 360 度旋转视频二维码

编号:**2009-15**

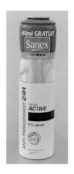

2009-15 号罐 360 度旋转视频二维码

编号:**2009-16**

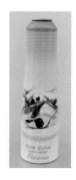

2009-16 号罐 360 度旋转视频二维码

十六、2008 年国际铝气雾罐竞赛参赛罐

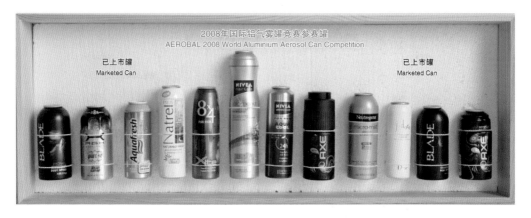

罐编号从左至右分别是:4,15,11,18,9,12,17,19,2,13,3,1

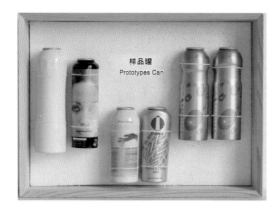

罐编号从左至右分别是:7,16,10,8,5,6

编号:2008-1

英文介绍

Can No. 1: Axe Dark Temptation Deodorant Body Spray

Marketed Can

Description: A combination of clear basecoat and translucent inks allow the rich bronze colours of the can to illuminate the flowing abstract design of the graphics on this container. The black ink, semi-matte over varnish and custom designed shoulder provide further dramatic impact to this modern design.

中文介绍

1号罐：

已上市罐

产品说明：

　　透明底涂层和半透明油墨的结合,使罐体浓郁的青铜色与容器上流动的抽象图案相得益彰。黑色油墨、哑光光油和定制设计的肩部为这个现代化的设计增添了更加引人注目的效果。

2008-1号罐360度旋转视频二维码

编号：**2008-2**

英文介绍

Can No.2: Neutrogena Micro-Mist Airbrush Sunless Tan

Marketed Can

Description: The graphic design of this can utilizes a special matched gold basecoat that provides an elegant look to the container. The crisp clean graphics provide eye appeal.

中文介绍

2号罐：

已上市罐

产品说明：

　　这款产品的图形设计采用了一种特殊的金色底涂层,赋予罐体优雅的外观。干净利落的图形设计增强了视觉吸引力。

2008-2号罐360度旋转视频二维码

编号：**2008-3**

英文介绍

Can No.3: Blade Diablo Deodorant Body Spray

Marketed Can

Description: The monochromatic colour scheme of this design in combination with

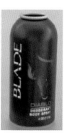

transparent ink over brushed aluminium creates the drama of a phantom image on this container. Further impact is achieved with crisp, clean, reversed text.

中文介绍

3 号罐：

已上市罐

产品说明：

这个设计的单色配色方案结合透明油墨在磨砂铝材,为这个罐体营造出一种幻影图像的戏剧艺术效果,清晰干净反向文字进一步增强了视觉冲击力。

2008-3 号罐 360 度旋转视频二维码

编号：**2008-4**

英文介绍

Can No. 4: Blade Howl Deodorant Body Spray

Marketed Can

Description: The fine brushing on the aluminium container utilizes the stark contrast

to the black ink background of these graphics, creating a stunning 3-dimensional holographic effect to this design. The container is further accented with crisp, "knocked out" text.

中文介绍

4 号罐：

已上市罐

产品说明：

铝制容器上的精细拉丝处理与黑色油墨背景形成鲜明对比,创造了令人惊叹的三维全息效果。容器还配以清晰的"镂空"文字达到引人注目的效果。

2008-4 号罐 360 度旋转视频二维码

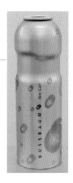

编号:2008-5

Can No. 5: Challenge Shape

Prototypes Can

Description:

First cver seen aluminium aerosol can asymmetrically shaped.

Based on a new shaping technology.

Handgrip with two disproportional bulges, which give the can a distinctive appearance.

Good handling by the integrated handgrip.

Ideal for shower gel and other products to be used in shower-bath and bath-tub.

A creative packaging for all product ranges, where shapes are used.

The asymmetric shape can be positioned exactly corresponding to the print design.

Available for 200 mL filling volume, other sizes will follow.

5 号罐:

样品罐

产品说明:

这是一款首次采用新型成型技术的非对称的铝气雾剂罐。

握柄处有两个不规则的凸出部位,使罐体有一个独特的外观。

得益于握柄的优化,使罐体有良好的抓握感。

适用于沐浴露等在浴室和浴缸中使用的产品。

适用于所有形状各异的创意的包装。

不对称的形状可以精确地与印刷设计匹配。

可用于 200 mL 的容量现已上市,其他规格的也将陆续推出。

2008-5号罐 360 度旋转视频二维码

编号:2008-6

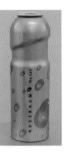

Can No. 6: Cosmos Shape

Prototypes Can

Description:

First ever seen aluminium aerosol can asymmetrically shaped.

Based on a new shaping technology.

Good handling by the special shape of the handgrip.

Ideal for shower gel and other products to be used in shower-bath and bath-tub.

A creative, distinctive and extraordinairy packaging for all product ranges, where shapes are used.

The asymmetric shape can be positioned exactly corresponding to the print design.

Available for 200 mL filling volume, other sizes will follow.

中文介绍

6 号罐:

样品罐

产品说明:

这是一款首次采用新型成型技术的非对称的铝气雾剂罐。

握柄处有两个不规则的凸出部位,使罐体有一个独特的外观。

得益于握柄的优化,使罐体有良好的抓握感。

适用于沐浴露等在浴室和浴缸中使用的产品。

适用于所有形状各异的创意的包装。

不对称的形状可以精确地与印刷设计匹配。

可用于 200 mL 的容量现已上市,其他规格的也将陆续推出。

2008-6 号罐 360 度旋转视频二维码

编号:2008-7

英文介绍

Can No. 7: Corona Shape

Prototypes Can

Description:

Combination of the soft, elegant "Evolution" shape with additional 12 angles at the-top of the can.

An attractive symbiosis of a smooth rather female shape and rather male shaping-elements: the angles.

The angles symbolise masculinity. So the can enhances a masculine image of the product.

Good handling by the reduced diameter in the middle of the can, like a grip shape.

Ideal for men's care products like shower gel, deo, shaving mousse, etc.

Ideal for technical products, which require a safe usage in hand.

A creative packaging for all product ranges, where masculinity should be supported.

Available for 200 to 250 mL filling volume, other sizes will follow.

中 文 介 绍

7 号罐:

样品罐

产品说明:

该款采用柔和优雅的"进化"造型与罐的顶部的 12 个角度相融合。

这是一种迷人的融合,将光滑的女性化形状与男性化的棱角元素相结合。

这些角度象征着男性气质,从而提升了产品的男性形象。

通过减少罐身中部的直径,使其具握把形状而便于抓握。

适合男性护理产品,如沐浴露、香体剂、剃须摩丝等。

适合需要以安全正确的握法使用的技术创新产品。

适合所有需要突显男性气质的产品创意包装。

目前适用于 200 mL 至 250 mL 的产品,其他容量罐体也将陆续推出。

2008-7 号罐 360 度旋转视频二维码

编号:2008-8

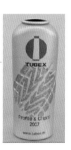

英 文 介 绍

Can No. 8: Profile & Grip(s)

Prototypes Can

Description: This can is special. It is shaped and debossed.

The print is orientated to the oval can with the round bottom and the debossing is also orientated to the print.

The new ergonomic and innovative oval design of the aerosol container is a synonym for technology expressed through its shape. The aerosol container is haptic convenient, conveys high quality and has a distinctive can design for maximum customer recognition due to improved shelf impression.

The debossing of the can is done inline. The process allows debossing of outlines as well as whole fields.

The aluminium aerosol can additionally reaches a considerable upgrading in respect of haptic and optic.

Debossing, which is possible over the whole can surface, creates a totally new, unmistakable tactile feeling.

Further important advantages of this prodedure are the high brand recognition of the consumer and as well the better protection against plagiarism.

中文介绍

8号罐:

样品罐

产品说明:

这款气雾剂罐很特别。它的形状和凹凸设计相得益彰。

图案面向具有圆形底的椭圆形罐,凹凸设计也朝向图案。

这种创新的符合人体工程学的椭圆形气雾剂罐设计可以通过其造型来表达它的技术感。气雾剂罐方便携带,传达出高品质,而且设计独特,能够提升其货架展示效果,最大程度获得客户的认可。

罐子的凹凸工艺是在线完成。整个过程允许对轮廓和整个区域进行凹凸设计。

铝气雾剂罐在触觉和视觉方面也得到了显著提升。

可在整个罐体表面进行凹凸设计的工艺,创造出全新的无可争议的触觉感受。

这种工艺的另一个重要优点是消费者对品牌的高度认可,具有更好的防伪保护作用。

2008-8号罐360度旋转视频二维码

编号:2008-9

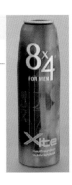

英文介绍

Can No. 9: 8×4 Xite

Marketed Can

Description: This is a special edition from the 8×4 range.

The shape is especially developed for a customer in order to differentiate. The special form gives the can a unique face. The can impresses with a clear and straightforward shape and gives the brand an unmistakable face.

The brushed can is printed with a combination of translucent and full-tone colours (7 colours) and has very fine screens (combination of frequency modulated screen and conventional screen) which shows changeable effects. The semi-mat over varnish completes the design. The challenge is to guarantee reproduction of the effects during the industrial production. With its technical/graphical print design the can is specially made for men.

中 文 介 绍

9 号罐：

已上市罐

产品说明：

这是 8×4 系列的特别版。

该款罐的形状是专门为客户设计的，以使其与众不同。特殊的形状使罐子具有独特的外观。罐子以其清晰而简洁的形状给人留下深刻印象，使品牌拥有独特的外观。

磨砂罐采用透明和全色调的 7 种颜色印刷，具有非常精细的视面（调制印版和常规印版的结合），通过半哑光光油完成，呈现多变的效果。其挑战在于确保在工业生产过程中复制这种效果。凭借其技术/图案印刷设计，该罐特别适合男性。

2008-9 号罐 360 度旋转视频二维码

编号：**2008-10**

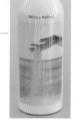

英 文 介 绍

Can No. 10: What a Feeling

Prototypes Can

Description: The upgrading of the standard can is done by a special haptical (partial) effect on the can surface—you can feel the sand (or other materials like ie. rubber, velvet etc.)! This is possible for serial production and available from rough to soft, from mat to gloss. This new effect intensifies the visual impression of the design and offers new possibilities for marketing/designers.

中 文 介 绍

10 号罐：

样品罐

产品说明：

罐体标准的升级可以通过在罐体表面施加特殊的触觉效果来实现——你可以感受到沙

子或其他材料,比如橡胶、天鹅绒等。这种效果可以在批量生产中实现,从粗糙到柔软、从哑光到高光均可选择。这种新的效果可以增强设计视觉效果,为市场营销和设计师提供新的可能性。

2008-10号罐360度旋转视频二维码

编号:2008-11

英文介绍

Can No. 11: Aquafresh

Marketed Can

Description: Totally new and innovative application: first toothpaste in an aerosol container. The can itself is a brushed can that shows metallic effects by using translucent print colours. The rays are being achieved by two different white tones that run into each other. The blank aluminium twinkles out of the printed toothpaste and conveys a bright smile. The real innovation—the internal powder coating—is invisible to the consumer, inside the aerosol can itself. Powder coating can be used in serial production now. This varnish is free of solvents and causes no emissions (no afterburner used, no CO_2 emissions).

This is technological break-through to environment-friendly production of aluminium aerosol cans in terms of internal coating. It has a very economic use of resources (re-use of overspray possible) and this coating has same (or better) characteristics as existing coatings. The internal powder coating is applied on modified standard production lines for aerosol cans.

中文介绍

11号罐:

已上市罐

产品说明:

这是全新和创新的应用:首次将牙膏装入喷雾容器中。罐子本身是一个拉丝抛光罐,通过使用半透明的油墨印刷展示其金属效果。由两种不同的白色色调相互交织产生了光芒的效果。空白的铝制表面反射出印在牙膏上的图案,传达出明亮的笑容。真正的创新之处在于罐体内部的粉末涂层,它在喷雾罐内部是看不见的。粉末涂层现已可用于批量生产。这种涂层不含溶剂,不会产生排放,无需使用后燃室,也不会产生二氧化碳排放。

这是在铝制喷雾罐内部涂层方面实现环保生产的技术突破。它在资源利用方面具有很高的经济效益,可以回收过喷的材料,而且这种涂层具有与现有涂层相同或更好的特性。内部粉末涂层是在经过改造的标准喷雾罐生产线上应用的。

2008-11 号罐 360 度旋转视频二维码

编号:2008-12

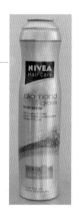

英 文 介 绍 ─────────────

Can No. 12: Nivea Hair Care Diamond Gloss

Marketed Can

Description: The can impresses with the extreme shaping and the excellent product decoration. The unique shape is specially developed for our customer in order to differentiate. Due to the immense waist the standard length has to be extended in order to achieve the filling volume. Therefore the can looks more slim, is a real "eye-catcher" on the shelf (standard length for 250 mm cans exceeded) and very convenient to handle. There is a smooth transition from the original diameter to the waist of the can which continues up to the shoulder. The special shape combines strong recession in the waist area and widening in the round-edged shoulder. The print itself also is a big challenge in order to bring the logo in the desired design after shaping. The smooth surface is achieved by a special aluminium alloy and necking technology. The diamond gloss effect is achieved by a combination of a pearlescent base coat (special pigment) and a transparent glossy over varnish. It is also supported by the harmonious mix of full-tone and translucent print colours with fine screens.

中 文 介 绍 ─────────────

12 号罐:

已上市罐

产品说明:

该罐以极致的造型和卓越的产品装饰给人留下深刻的印象。独特的形状是专门为我们的客户设计的,以使其与众不同。由于腰部的极度收缩,标准长度必须延长,以达到所需的填充容量。因此,罐子看起来很纤细,在货架上非常"引人注目"(标准长度超过 250 mm 的范围),并且非常方便抓握。罐体有一个平滑的过渡,从原始直径到腰再延续到肩部。这种特殊的形状结合了腰部的强烈收缩和肩部的圆润扩展。印刷本身也是一个很大的挑战,需要在成型后将徽标完美地呈现出来。平滑的表面是通过特殊的铝合金和缩颈技术来实现的。钻石亮光效果是通过珠光底涂层(特殊颜料)和透明光油的组合实现的。全色调和半透明印刷色彩与精细印刷的完美结合为其提供了支持。

2008-12 号罐 360 度旋转视频二维码

编号：**2008-13**

英文介绍

Can No. 13: J'adore

Marketed Can

Description: J'adore artwork is an example mixing elegance, sobriety, purity and finesse. This artwork is 100% achieved with hot stamping. The artwork background does not allow any drift. The contrast between the mat over varnish and the golden gloss of hot stamping is eye catching. The soft touch provides a great feeling while held in hand.

中文介绍

13 号罐：

已上市罐

产品说明：

J'adore 图案融合了优雅、简洁、纯洁和精巧。这幅图案是通过 100% 烫印技术实现的。图案背景不允许任何偏差。哑光表面和金色亮光烫印之间的对比非常引人注目。当握在手中时，柔软的触感提供了一种无与伦比的感觉。

2008-13 号罐 360 度旋转视频二维码

编号：**2008-15**

英文介绍

Can No. 15: RGX Pure 50 Body Spray

Marketed Can

Description: The elegance of the brushed aluminium container radiates through the soft metallic ink to create an enchanting ghosted tattoo effect on this container. The demur shades of the lower background graphics have a subtle fade to black in the embossed/debossed area of the can which provides dramatic impact on this modern, masculine design.

中 文 介 绍

15 号罐：

已上市罐

产品说明：

　　拉丝抛光铝罐的优雅可以通过柔和的金属油墨散发出来，在罐体上创造出迷人的幻影文身效果。背景图形的暗色调在罐体的浮雕/凹面浮雕区域有一种微妙的黑色渐变，为这种具有现代气息的、男性化的设计带来了巨大的影响。

2008-15 号罐 360 度旋转视频二维码

编号：**2008-16**

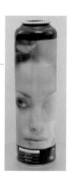

英 文 介 绍

Can No. 16: High Definition Four Colour Printing Prototypes Can

Description: Following demand from the aerosol market and its customers for improved printing quality and aesthetics on aluminium aerosol cans, Boxal has developed high definition printing which leads to unprecedented quality in printing aluminium aerosol cans.

The prototype can is printed in CMYK/4C colours which opens up more opportunitiesfor differentiation in design and more complex designs. This was up to now not possible in the printing of aluminium aerosols.

High definition printing presents opportunities to come extremely close to photo-realistic printing results using conventional dry offset printing methods. Screen colours can fade out to almost 0, eliminating a cut-off upon reaching the minimum dot size.

High definition printing also opens up possibilities to reduce the font size which can lead to more text on same area on the back-of-pack, more country variant texts could be printed on the aerosol back-of-pack.

中 文 介 绍

16 号罐：

样品罐

产品说明：

　　应气雾剂市场和客户对铝气雾剂罐改进印刷质量和提升美观的更高要求，Boxal 开发了高清晰度印刷技术，从而实现了铝气雾剂罐前所未有的印刷质量。

该样品罐以 CMYK/4C 颜色印刷，为设计的差异化和更复杂的设计提供了更多的可能性。到目前为止，这种技术在铝制气雾剂罐的印刷中是不可能实现的。

高清晰度印刷技术使用传统的干胶印刷方法，非常接近逼真的印刷效果。网点颜色可以渐变到几乎为 0，从而消除了达到最小网点尺寸时的限制。

高清印刷还为减小字体大小提供了可能性，这可以在相同区域的罐背上打印更多的文本。还可以在喷雾剂罐背上打印更多的国家版本的文本。

2008-16 号罐 360 度旋转视频二维码

编号：2008-17

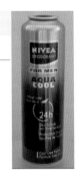

英文介绍

Can No. 17: Nivea

Marketed Can

Description: In an effort to respond to the aerosol market's demand for reduction of the environmental impact of aerosols, Boxal has developed water based base and o-ver varnish lacquers for aerosols.

In close cooperation with Beiersdorf, the development of water based lacquers is made, not losing or rather even improving the aesthetical aspects of the cans and their printing/design.

Leading to a reduction in emissions from Boxal factories and improving particularly the glossy properties of the cans, Nivea cans are now produced with water based lacquers.

Boxal will implement water based lacquers on its complete range of aerosols. This leads to a substantial reduction in emission in Boxal production sites. This is a significant step in supporting environmental improvement efforts by both Boxal and its customers.

中文介绍

17 号罐：

已上市罐

产品说明：

为了响应气雾剂市场对减少环境影响的需求，Boxal 开发了用于气雾剂罐的水性底涂层和水性光油。

在与 Beiersdorf 的密切合作下，公司开发了水性光油，不仅没有失去甚至提高了罐体及其印刷设计的美学效果。

为了减少 Boxal 工厂的排放，特别是提高了罐体的光泽度，妮维雅气雾罐现在都使用水性光油生产。

Boxal 将在其全系列的气雾剂罐上使用水性光油。这将使 Boxal 的生产基地排放大幅减少。这是 Boxal 及其客户支持环境改善的重要一步。

2008-17 号罐 360 度旋转视频二维码

编号：**2008-18**

英 文 介 绍

Can No. 18: Natrel

Marketed Can

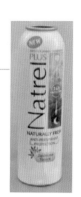

Description: In close cooperation with Schwarzkopf & Henkel, Boxal has launched production of Natrel cans with high definition printing utilising CMYK/4C. High definition printing aspects of the design are best shown in the visual of the Natrel aerosol cans. This represents the first industrial realisation of CMYK/4P on aluminium aerosol cans in dry offset.

High definition printing improves printing quality and aesthetics on aluminium aerosol cans.

中 文 介 绍

18 号罐：

已上市罐

产品说明：

在与 Schwarzkopf & Henkel 的密切合作下，Boxal 推出了利用 CMYK/4C 高清晰度印刷的 Natrel 气雾剂罐。设计的高清晰度印刷外观在 Natrel 气雾剂罐视觉效果中得到了最好的展示。这代表了 CMYK/4P 在干胶印制铝气雾罐上的首次工业应用。

高清晰度印刷技术提高了铝气雾剂罐的印刷质量和美感。

2008-18 号罐 360 度旋转视频二维码

编号:2008-19

英 文 介 绍

Can No. 19: AXE Dark Temptation

Marketed Can

Description: The artwork for "AXE Dark Temptation" has been a real challenge for the technical teams. They have to translate the brand spirit (deodorant that makes you feel irresistible) while enhancing the sweetness and silkiness of hot chocolate. Beyond the brand identity the logo they have to work on printing frames, inks and also over varnish to ensure an effect on the can as expected by the customer. The commercial success of the global launch is worth all the efforts that are involved in setting up this artwork, and the roof that they are able to achieve this type of challenge by applying all their know-how and latest printing techniques.

中 文 介 绍

19 号罐:

已上市罐

产品说明:

"AXE Dark Temptation" 的图案设计对技术团队来说是一个真正的挑战。他们必须在提升热巧克力的甜度和丝滑感的同时,诠释品牌精神(让你感到无法抗拒的香体剂)。除了品牌标识之外,他们还必须在印刷框架、油墨和光油上进行细致的工作,确保罐体上的效果符合客户的预期。全球推出的这款产品所取得的商业成功证明了他们在设计这一艺术作品时所付出的努力是值得的,也证明了他们能够通过他们自己的全部专业知识和最新的印刷技术来应对这类挑战。

2008-19 号罐 360 度旋转视频二维码

2

第二篇
国际特色马口铁气雾罐

国际特色马口铁气雾罐及视频

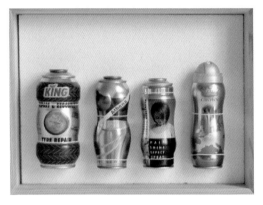

产品编号从左至右分别是:530,506,519,554

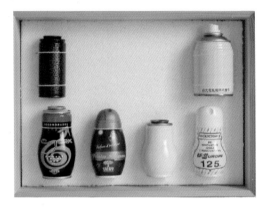

产品编号从左至右分别是:545,524,504,503,502,501

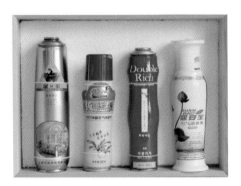

产品编号从左至右分别是:515,511,544,516

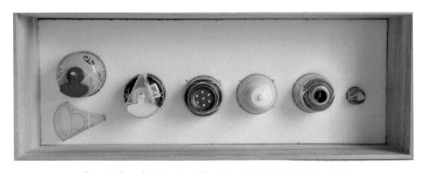

产品编号从左至右分别是:546,547,548,520,514,526

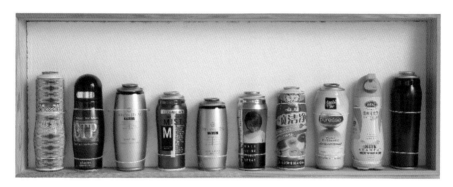

产品编号从左至右分别是:509,512,517,505,523,518,536,513,508,510

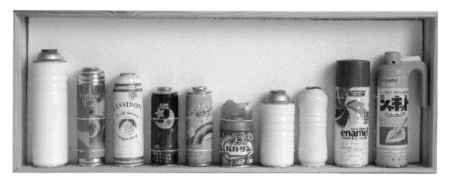

产品编号从左至右分别是:542,534,555,558,557,539,540,533,541,543

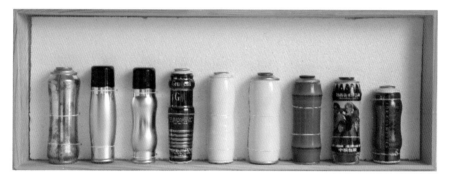

产品编号从左至右分别是:553,538,529,527,535,552,525,522,507

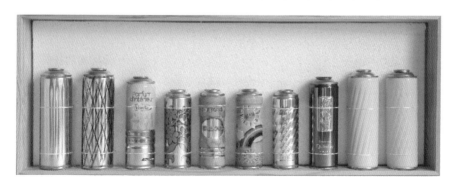

产品编号从左至右分别是:549,528,537,556,532,531,521,559,550,551

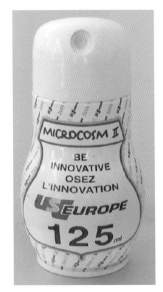

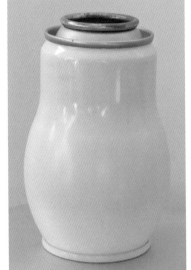

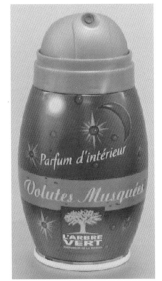

501

502

503

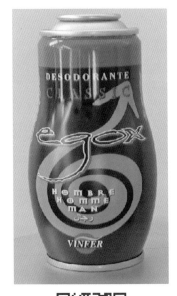

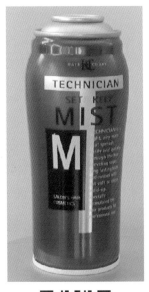

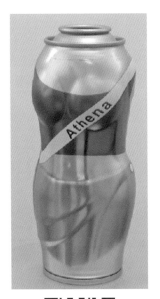

504

505

506

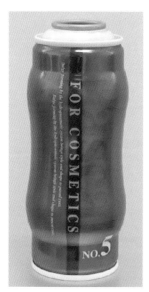

507

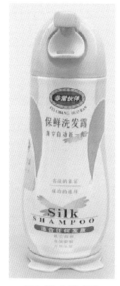

508

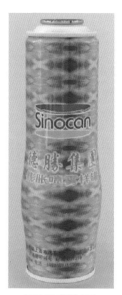

509

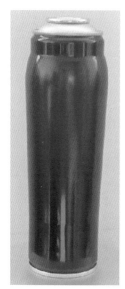

510

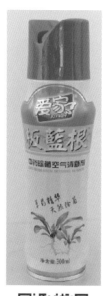

511

512

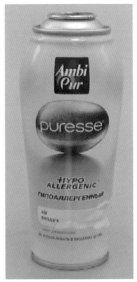

513

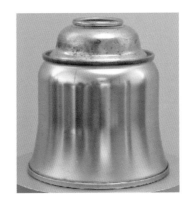

514

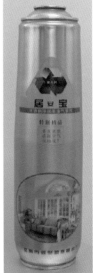

515

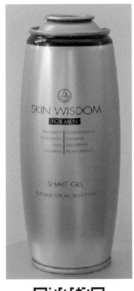

516

517

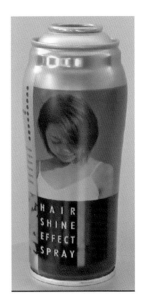

518

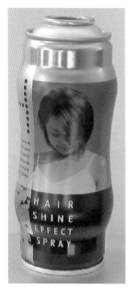

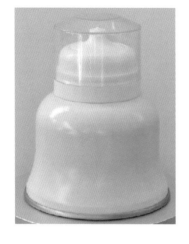

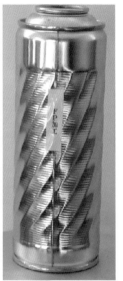

519

520

521

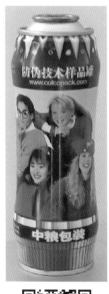

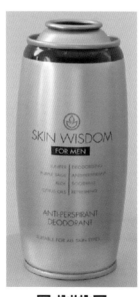

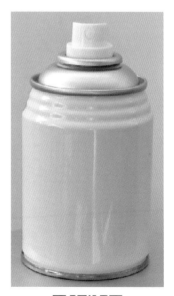

522

523

524

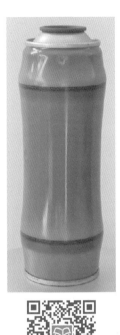

525

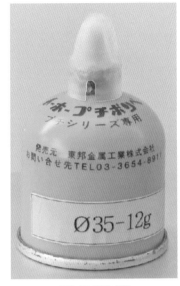

526

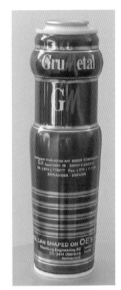

527

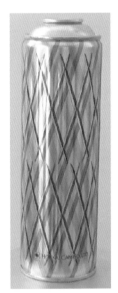

528

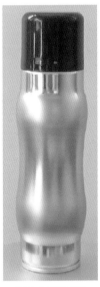

529

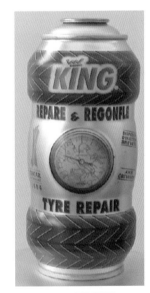

530

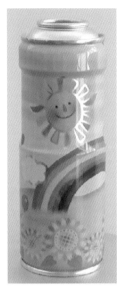

531

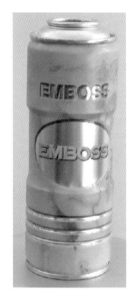

532

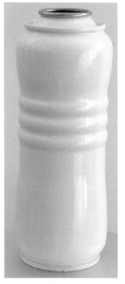

533

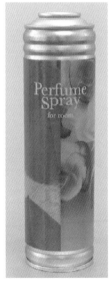

534

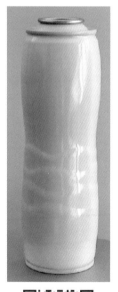

535

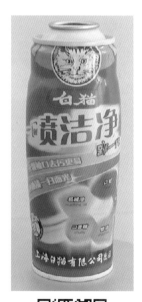

536

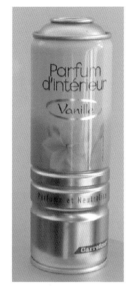

537

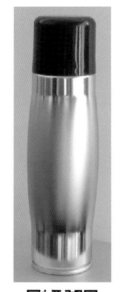

538

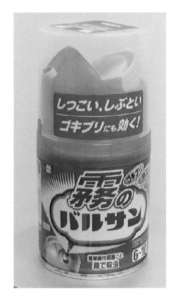

539

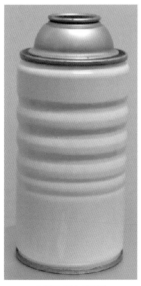

540

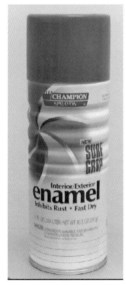

541

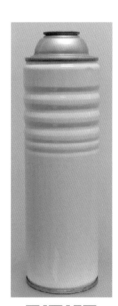

542

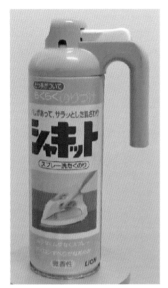

543

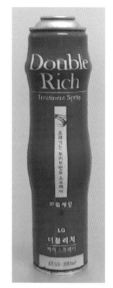

544

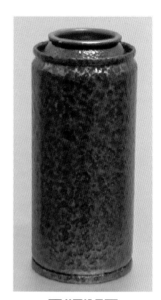

545

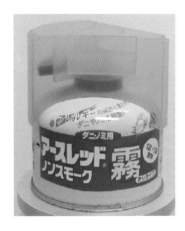

546

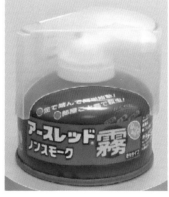

547

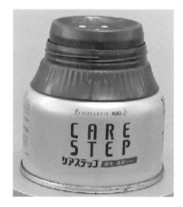

548

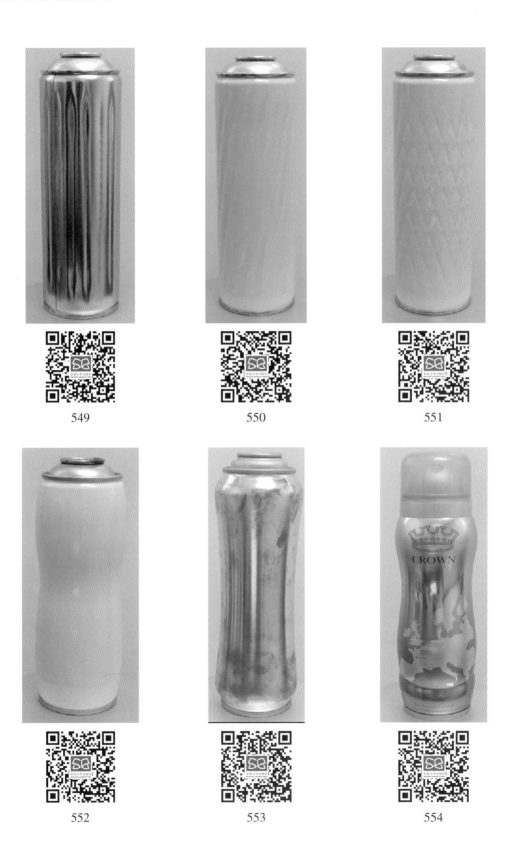

549

550

551

552

553

554

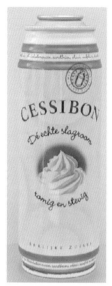

555

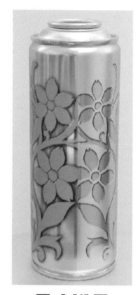

556

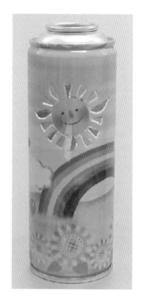

557

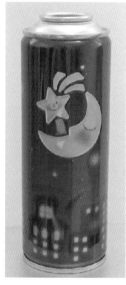

558

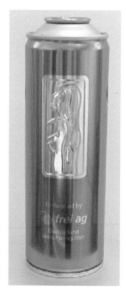

559